D0003372

How to keep Healthy & Happy by Fasting

BY SALEM KIRBAN

Published by SALEM KIRBAN, Inc., Kent Road, Huntingdon Valley, Penna. 19006. Copyright © 1976 by Salem Kirban. Printed in the United States of America. All rights reserved, including the right to reproduce this book or portions thereof in any form.

Library of Congress Catalog Card No. 75-29586
ISBN 0-912582-23-5

Excerpts from
HOW TO KEEP HEALTHY and HAPPY by FASTING!

You will not feel hungry when you fast! I know . . . because I have tried it. Not only will you NOT feel hungry . . . but for once in your life . . . you will feel **ALIVE!**   chapter 1
* * *

In 46 B.C., Julius Caesar passed a law which placed a limit on the amount of money which might be spent on food.   chapter 2
* * *

Much of today's advertising uses what is termed subliminal seduction. The preparation of one minute commercials can run from $50,000 to as high as $250,000!   chapter 3
* * *

Americans are becoming a nation of processed, packaged and preserved people. With the junk foods we eat, we consume every year more than 4 pounds of chemical preservatives, stabilizers, colorings, flavorings and other additives.   chapter 4
* * *

Advertisers in the fast-food industry bombard us with clowns jumping around with hamburgers and french fries. And it would seem totally un-American not to patronize them.   chapter 5
* * *

Of the 28,000 medical books, only 4 books are listed under FASTING! Benjamin Franklin reminds us: *"He's the best physician that knows the worthlessness of most medicines."*   chapter 6
* * *

When you make your stomach a garbage can . . . your heart suffers, your arteries suffer, you poison your blood stream.   chapter 8
* * *

When you fast, you will not find it unusual to lose five pounds the first day!   chapter 9
* * *

Fasting gives a complete rest from the digestive processes so the organs of the body can devote their energies of self-healing and self-rejuvenation.   chapter 10
* * *

If you and your wife fast one day a week, you will save money, by not eating 156 meals a year. Those who have tried it say they look and feel younger, rarely have headaches and colds, lose excess weight and have a happier marriage.   chapter 11
* * *

Most people have found out that short 24-hour fasts will achieve as great or greater benefits than long fasts!   chapter 12
* * *

Fasting can be the beginning of a new and better life for you! chapter 14
* * *

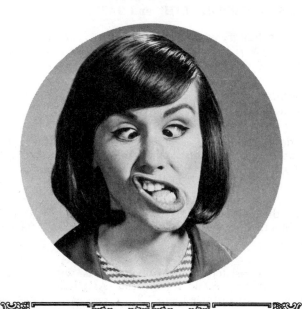

WHAT! ME FAST?
YOU MUST BE CRAZY?
I'D DIE OF STARVATION!
I COULDN'T EXIST IF I MISSED ONE
MEAL!

(If reading a book on fasting
causes a reaction
like the young lady pictured
then
THIS BOOK IS FOR YOU!
I dare you to read it!
It can change your life
    for the better!

Fasting is **not** starving. And short, periodic fasts may start you on the road to better health and a longer and happier life!)

DEDICATION

My wife
MARY

"Who can find a virtuous woman?

For her price is far above rubies.

A virtuous woman is a crown to her husband. . ."

(Proverbs 31:10; 12:4)

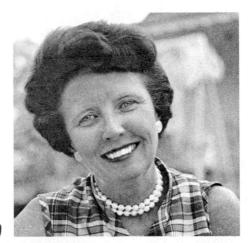

My wife, Mary.
Her life is a constant inspiration to me.

It was Mary who first brought the idea of fasting to my attention. And I can't thank her enough for it. Since then, each of us fasts one day each week. And it has given us a vibrancy we have never known before. (I believe she is getting younger every day!)

Sacrifice and dedication are the words that best describe Mary. While I was going through college, she even sold auto parts to gas stations so we could make ends meet. In our early years of marriage she overlooked my insufficiencies and nurtured our 5 children in a home that was and is Christ-centered. It was only in 1968 that I began writing books. (One might say my first 40 years were spent in the "wilderness.")

Her life is her Christian testimony. Her life is a constant inspiration to me. And my books have become a reality because of her continual encouragement bathed in a foundation of prayer.

ACKNOWLEDGMENTS

To **Dr. Gary G. Cohen,** Professor of Greek and New Testament at Biblical School of Theology, Hatfield, Pa., who carefully checked the final manuscript.

To **Doreen Frick,** who carefully proofread the text.

To **Diane Kirban,** who created the chart on those in Scripture who fasted.

To **Bob Krauss,** artist, who designed the front cover and coordinated all the art work.

To **Edston Detrich** and **Paul Benedetti,** who designed the back cover.

To **Walter W. Slotilock,** Chapel Hill Litho, for skillfully making all the illustration negatives.

To **Batsch Company** for excellent craftsmanship in setting the type.

To **Dickinson Brothers, Inc.,** for printing with all possible speed and quality.

Scriptures used include the King James Version of the Bible and The New American Standard Bible (ASV) By Permission of the Lockman Foundation.

CONTENTS

Note

This book was written to introduce you to the concept of fasting. Those who have conducted fasting clinics, supervising some 30,000 to 50,000 fasts, have found that fasting has a beneficial effect for physical and mental problems.

Those individuals who fast periodically, including well-known personalities and those in the medical profession also report beneficial results.

However, nothing in this book is intended to constitute medical treatment or advice of any nature.

Moreover, it is recommended that before any person fasts, one should visit his doctor for initial and continued supervision.

Salem Kirban

WHY I WROTE THIS BOOK

I am appalled at the number of people who ignore all the natural laws of nutrition and living. . .
and then expect their doctor to work a miracle in their lives!
I am appalled at the number of people who pour into their body a conglomerate of munchies, crunchies and french fries. . .
and then expect God to heal them!

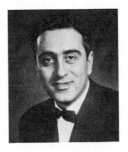

I am appalled at the number of medical men who believe that today's buffered, preserved, antioxidanted, emulsified, sequestranted, stabilized, bleached, texturized and methyl salicylated food is sufficient to maintain good health.

I am appalled at the number of doctors who believe the simple commonsense solutions are antiquated and drugs and surgery the best answer.

I am appalled at the number of doctors who are more concerned about the **cure** of illness rather than the **prevention!**

This book is cheaper than a visit to your doctor. Yet most people would rather spend money after they become sick than exercise common sense and learn how their body works, and how to keep it well!

You can't pour junk into the miracle that God has given to you — your body — and expect to keep healthy and happy. But that's exactly what you do when you eat junk foods, loaded with preservatives and additives and ingest so-called miracle drugs. If we obey the laws of God, we can share in the gifts of God.

It's time for a change!

That's why I wrote this book!

Salem Kirban

Huntingdon Valley, Pennsylvania
U.S.A., November, 1975

1

GO WITHOUT FOOD ? PERISH THE THOUGHT!

**Americans
are
Food-oriented**

Americans have been so bombarded with television commercials from fast-food drive-ins . . that to think for one minute of skipping a meal almost borders on being unpatriotic!

We are food-oriented. And we actually believe that it is necessary for us to have 3 square meals a day. We pride ourself on having fat babies and wouldn't think of skipping breakfast!

We are so grateful that we live in the land of Shake 'n Bake bags and can cook our food in sturdy plastic containers.

Everything we seem to do in America is ON THE RUN. We eat on the run . . . and die on the run.

Our economy and much of our advertising is based on the fact that happiness can only come from material success in life . . . those extra accessories on the car . . . the ability to "have it your way" when ordering your fat-saturated hamburger . . . the thrill of "smoking for taste and not for tar."

Most doctors are oriented to treating illnesses rather than preventing them! And while they excise a diseased lung in the operating room . . . their hospital is still often selling cigarettes in the gift shop.

Airlines will not tolerate a hijacker . . . for fear of taking the other passengers a few thousand miles out of their way on an exodus to Cuba. And they spend millions of dollars daily in anti-hijacking devices and security personnel to make sure a hijacking does not occur. YET, they allow people to smoke in airplanes (in a section they call a smoking section) which poisons the entire cabin atmosphere with pollutants which can only contribute to ill health!

What a paradox!

It was Benjamin Franklin who said:

> I saw few die of hunger,
> of eating − 100,000.

The Talmud tells us:

> In eating, a third of the stomach should be filled with food . . . a third with drink, and the rest left empty.

More people are killed by over-eating and drinking than by wars!

Tell me what you eat and I'll tell you what you are!

There is a well-known saying that:

> The way to a man's heart
> is through his stomach.

And how true this is. Many wives have perhaps unknowingly, by overstuffing their husband with junk foods and sweet pastries, have generated business for their local undertaker quicker than he anticipated!

Most everyone likes to eat . . . but few people know when to stop. No man in the world has more courage than the man who can stop after eating one peanut.

Someone once said:

> *Hunger is not only the best cook, but also the best physician!*

Most people when they first hear about fasting . . . laugh in ridicule and say:

> *I could never fast. I would starve! I would die of hunger!*

In this book, I may repeat myself on this one particular point . . . because many people find it difficult to understand.

YOU WILL NOT FEEL HUNGRY WHEN YOU FAST!

I know . . . because I have tried it; as have countless thousands. Not only will you NOT feel hungry . . . but for once in your life . . . you will feel <u>ALIVE</u>!

But, right now, you are probably still saying:

> *Go without food? Perish the thought!*

You have the choice to make.

Go back to stuffing yourself at every meal . . . getting up from the table bloated and sleepy.

Wake up every morning feeling dull and dragged out and more tired than when you went to bed.

Go spend money at your doctor's office and come out with a prescription and take myriad variety of pills.

Your doctor is not God who alone can heal! And he will be the first to admit it. In fact, many doctors themselves are the worst offenders with poor eating and fasting habits.

Specialists and Physicians

It was Dr. William J. Mayo himself who said:

> A specialist is a man
> who knows more and more
> about less and less.

And Napoleon Bonaparte remarked:

> In my opinion physicians kill as many
> people as we generals.

Physicians are of all men most happy; what good success they have the world proclaims and what faults they commit the earth covers.

Will Rogers believed that the best doctor in the world is the veterinarian. He can't ask his patients what is the matter — he's just got to know.

Mark Twain humorously remarked:

> He has been a doctor a year now and
> has had two patients – no, three, I
> think – yes, it was three; I attended
> their funerals.

Doctors are not known for being in full

agreement with anything. In fact, I am sure many doctors will scoff at this book. The medical art is not so cut and dried that you cannot find some authority for doing whatever you please. If your doctor does not think it good for you to sleep, to drink, or to eat of a particular dish, do not worry; I will find you another who will not agree with him.

There is much truth in what Benjamin Franklin said:

God heals and the doctor takes the fee.

One would think by reading this that I do not like doctors. That is not true. To repeat a well-worn phrase:

Some of my best friends are doctors.

God has allowed doctors through the miracle of surgery to perform great services to humanity. Physicians are needed and should be respected. They have gone through 8-16 years of intensive training to study their profession.

Dr. Allan Cott, a knowledgeable doctor, who wrote the book, Fasting, The Ultimate Diet, said:

Fasting may be effective in treating many more varieties of sickness than orthodox medical circles are ever likely to concede.

I am dismayed by the number of my colleagues who brand all naturopaths and chiropractors and hygienists as "charlatans."

On the other hand, I am also turned off

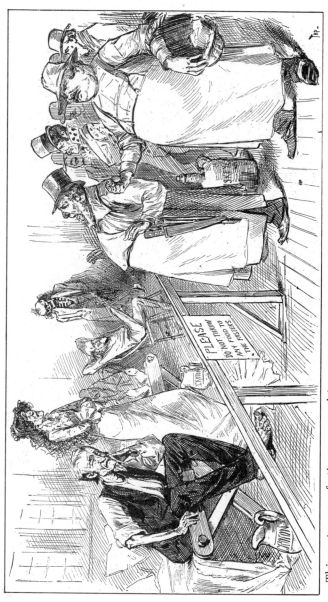

This cartoon on fasting appeared in an 1880 magazine. It is captioned: THE NEW CRAZE AND ITS CONSEQUENCES . . . Butchers, Bakers, and All: "*If this sort of thing continues, we'll all of us starve ourselves for want of business.*"

In the illustration those fasting are depicted as scrawny, ugly and dying. This attitude on fasting still prevails today.

*by the extreme "naturalists," who
claim the expertise of orthodox medicine is totally misguided.*
*Both groups have something to con-
tribute; they should be learning from
each other.*

I agree with Dr. Cott.

**The Value
of Rest**

In Genesis 2:2 we are told:

*And on the seventh day God ended His
work which He had made;
and He rested on the seventh day.*

My personal opinion — and here this is a
health opinion, not a theological one — is
that the body should follow this same
example. The digestive processes should
be given a rest . . . one day a week.

In a future chapter I will discuss what I
believe to be the ideal fast. I will also point
out some of the adverse effects that many
popular prescription drugs can have on the
human body.

It was Oliver Wendell Holmes who said:

*I firmly believe that if the whole
<u>materia medica</u> could be sunk to the
bottom of the sea, it would be all the
better for mankind and all the worse
for the fishes.*

Sir William Osler, a Canadian physician
and professor of medicine, said:

*One of the first duties of the physician
is to educate the masses <u>not</u> to take
medicine!*

Many believe the art of medicine consists
of amusing the patient while nature cures
the disease.

Health Aide Raps 'Burger Binge'

Pennsylvania Health Secretary Dr. Leonard Bachman feels fast food chains with their hamburgers, french fries and Cokes are breaking up American families and ruining their health.

"It is ironic, but as we observe our 200th anniversary we find new national shrines with such names as McDonald's, Burger King, Gino's, Colonel Sanders and Hardee's," Bachman told a meeting of Pennsylvania nutritionists in Harrisburg recently.

"The American staple has become the hamburger, followed closely by a large Coke and a side order of fries," he said. "The family mealtime has been replaced by individual snack time. Even the traditional family Sunday dinner is vanishing from American homes."

Dr. Bachman said there was an abysmal consumer ignorance on the subject of nutrition" and he blamed health professionals for failing + ∼+

their message through to the public. "We have not communicated our knowledge of the importance of a well-balanced diet to one's health," he said. "On the other hand, the fast food chains have bombarded the American public with such come-ons as 'Hold the pickle, hold the lettuce, special orders don't upset us. All we ask is that you let us serve you your way.'"

"The other harm is that a hamburger and fries at a fast food restaurant have replaced the evening meal for many families. That's the one meal when the whole family sits down together and interacts, and it's very important in keeping the family together.

"Without that necessary interaction of the mother and father and children you have families breaking up. And any number of health problems can be traced to the breakdown of the family."

TV snacks—yes, firm develops shape, taste

By   Food Technology people have developed a simulated potato skin which, when combined with dehydrated mashed potatoes, makes a quick and tasty baked potato.

Modern America appears too sophisticated to simply eat a farm-grown potato as God has given it to us. Instead we must remove the vitamin and mineral rich potato skin, mash the potato, dehydrate it, then develop a *simulated* or imitation skin! No wonder hospitals are filled!

**Health
is
Wealth**

During the depression of the 1930's my family was on welfare. As a lad of 8 and 9, we grew a garden and had to eat unpreserved foods from it. We could not afford candy bars. Instead we would chew on a rhubarb or a carrot.

And believe it or not . . . we had no TV. It hadn't been invented yet! So for enjoyment . . . my mother and sister and I would rock on the swing that we hung between two trees — the world's best tranquilizer.

And while I rarely even saw a penny (my mother once gave me a whole dime for Christmas) . . . we were happy and healthy. Down the road apiece was a typical country store. It sold everything from gasoline, nails, mousetraps and candy. I can remember begging my mother for one cent to buy a candy bar one hot summer day. She most always refused.

And my mother, in her broken Lebanese-English accent, would say,

Son, HEALTH IS WEALTH

How true that is!

Health is a crown on a well man's head, but no one can see it but a sick man.

How is your crown? Is it frayed, tarnished and starting to fall apart? Don't depend on your doctor to put it back together again. Go without food? Perish the thought!

Just this once . . . learn how going without food on a fast . . . may start you down a road of health and happiness you never thought possible!

2

FESTIVALS OF FEASTING

**A Dinner
of
40 Courses**

Three meals a day are a highly advanced institution. Savages of yesterday either gorged themselves or fasted.

Cannibalism at one time was found in nearly all primitive tribes. Human flesh was a staple item, funerals were rare. On the island of New Britain human meat was sold in shops as butcher's meat is sold.

Wil Durant, in his book, Our Oriental Heritage, reports:

> ... in some of the Solomon Islands, human victims, preferably women, were fattened for a feast like pigs... In Tahiti an old Polynesian chief explained his diet to Pierre Loti: "The white man, when well roasted, tastes like a ripe banana."
>
> The Fijians, however, complained that the flesh of the whites was too salty and tough.

The Chinese loved to eat and it was not unusual for a rich man's dinner to have over 40 courses and to require three or four hours to consume. American Presidents who have visited China even today find the Chinese dinners overwhelming.

At every possible moment of the year it seemed that the Greeks created a religious feast and festival to celebrate some occasion or other.

Not to be outdone, the Romans at one time had as many as 76 festivals a year. The rich Roman dined in his dining room which usually contained three couches. Each couch accommodated three people. The diner rested his head on his left arm, and his arm on a cushion. His body extended diagonally away from the serving table.

Canary a la King

The banquet began at four and lasted till late in the night or till the next day! To satisfy their educated tastes they ate rare fish, rare birds, rare fruit . . . some of which cost $40 a pound! Favorite dishes included:

the wings of ostriches
the tongues of flamingoes
the flesh of canaries

After the dinner, the diner emptied his stomach with an emetic. But some gluttons performed this operation during their meal, and then returned to the table to appease their hunger.

It was Seneca who said:

They vomit to eat,
and eat to vomit.

This practice was not typical, however of

all Roman eating, fortunately.

Prior to the great festival banquets the Romans revelled in gladiator games. There was even a professional gladiator school. Training and discipline were rigorous. Physicians made sure they ate barley to develop muscle. If they violated their diet, they were punished by scourging and confinement in chains!

However, on the eve of their combat they were given a rich banquet. Seneca was so moved by the wholesale slaughter of the gladiator combats that he wrote:

> *I am come home more greedy, more cruel and inhuman, because I have been among human beings.*
>
> *In the morning they throw men to the lions; at noon they throw them to the spectators.*
>
> *Man, a sacred thing to man, is killed for sport and merriment.*

In a more refined sense such inhumanity to man still continues today . . . and through many indiscretions in the food he eats he leads himself to an early grave.

It is a fact that the Romans were very fond of food. Men in those days squandered their fortunes on food . . . sometimes to the point of bankruptcy. To continue eating, they signed on as gladiators, knowing they would be well-fed at government expense.

The $40,000 Dinner

M. Gavius Apicius, who lived in the time of Tiberius Caesar, was a wealthy glutton. It has been said that after he spent about $4 million on food, he checked his accounts, and finding himself left with but a mere $400,000, committed suicide.

One Roman, shocked at the obsession with food, wrote:

> Intent on stuffing themselves, they follow their noses and the shrieking women's voices to the kitchen, and like a flock of starving and screeching peacocks they stand on the tips of their toes biting their finger-nails waiting for the food to cool.

It was not unusual for a festival dinner in the early Roman empire to cost $40,000!

A Law Limiting Food Purchase

In 46 B.C., Julius Caesar passed a law which placed a limit on the amount of money which might be spent on food. The law did not prove effective.

Drinking before dinner was a common practice even in Roman days.

Romans in the high social class ate in a reclining position. Affluent Romans were, after the dinner, carried home in a litter or a chair.

During the dinner the guests customarily threw objects of food which they discarded to the ground—legs of lobsters, shells of snails, egg shells, cherry stones or apple cores.

It is interesting to note that Romans ate little or no breakfast.

Many ate only one meal a day . . . stuffing themselves at noon.

No wonder Cicero wrote:

> Eat to live, not live to eat.

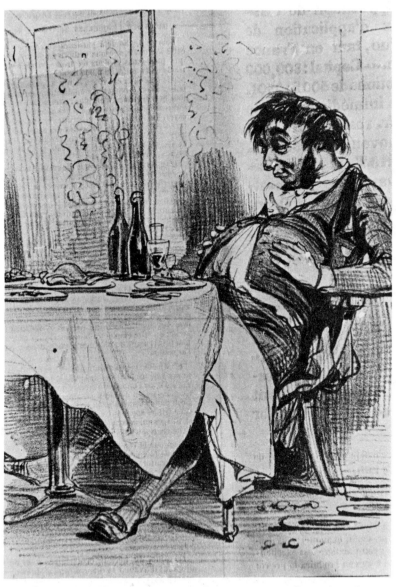

Are you eating your way to an early "retirement" from this planet? Could this illustration of a gourmet in 1838 also be a picture of your excesses?

**The Bible
on
Gluttony**

In the Bible, gluttony (excessive appetite) is characteristic of the wicked:

For many walk, of whom I (Paul) often told you, and now tell you even weeping, that they are enemies of the cross of Christ,

*whose end is destruction,
whose god is their appetite,
and whose glory is in their shame,
who set their minds on earthly things.*
(Philippians 3:18-19)

In the 10th century B.C., the God-inspired writer of Proverbs wrote:

*Listen, my son, and be wise,
And direct your heart in the way.
Do not be with heavy drinkers of wine,
Or with gluttonous eaters of meat;
For the heavy drinker and the glutton
  will come to poverty.*
(Proverbs 23:19-21)

There are examples of good and bad feasting in the Bible. Here are a few:

**To Unify
the
Nation**

Prior to entering the Promised Land the Israelites were to destroy all their heathen altars and burn the shameful images.

They then were reminded that when they entered the Promised Land they were to bring their tithes and their burnt offerings and the first-born of their herd and of their flock to a place chosen by the Lord (Shiloh, then Jerusalem).

There also you and your households shall eat before the Lord your God, and rejoice in all your undertakings in which the Lord your God has blessed you.

> You shall not do at all what we are
> doing here today, every man doing
> whatever is right in his own eyes.
> (Deuteronomy 12:7-8)

The Israelites had three annual feasts: the Passover, Pentecost and the Feast of the Tabernacle.

At the Lord's Supper

The Corinthian Christians conducted their meetings like some church business meetings of today. They were constantly arguing. Paul, in directing the saints in what is proper said:

> Therefore when you meet together, it is
> not to eat the Lord's Supper . . .

He then tells them:

> In your eating one takes his own sup-
> per first; and one is hungry and an-
> other is drunk.
> Do you not have houses in which to eat
> and drink? . . .
> (1 Corinthians 11:20-22)

He then reminds the Corinthians that in the house of the Lord they should remember the Lord's sacrifice for our sins and the promise that He is coming again.

Sad to say, many churches these days are filled with people who devote more time in the kitchen or banquet hall than in the sanctuary.

Jeroboam's Counterfeit Feast

When Solomon died, his son Rehoboam became ruler. Fearful of what they feared would be a harsh rule under Rehoboam, all the tribes except Judah deserted him and pledged their allegiance to Jeroboam.

Jeroboam was a rebel leader whom Solomon tried to kill (I Kings 11:40).

Jeroboam, fearful that the tribes he had won to his side might have second thoughts in their pilgrimage to Jerusalem, had two golden calf-idols made and set up in the cities of Dan and Bethel and told the people:

> It is too much for you to go up to Jerusalem; behold your gods, O Israel, that brought you up from the land of Egypt.
>
> (I Kings 12:28)

He also announced his own annual Tabernacle Festival in the eighth month. And Jeroboam's counterfeit feast led Israel into sin.

The Banquet of Ahasuerus

In the 5th Century B.C., the Jews were captives in Persia. Esther was a Jewish maiden who was to become queen of Persia and deliver her people from massacre. The King, Ahasuerus, was also called Xerxes, who reigned 486-465 B.C.

In the third year of his reign, he gave a banquet for all his princes and attendants, the army officers of Persia and Media, the nobles, and the princes of his provinces. See Esther 1.

For 180 days, 6 months, this celebration went on to provide a tremendous display of the wealth and glory of his empire.

When it was all over, the king decided to give a very special banquet; this time for the palace servants and officials alike. This

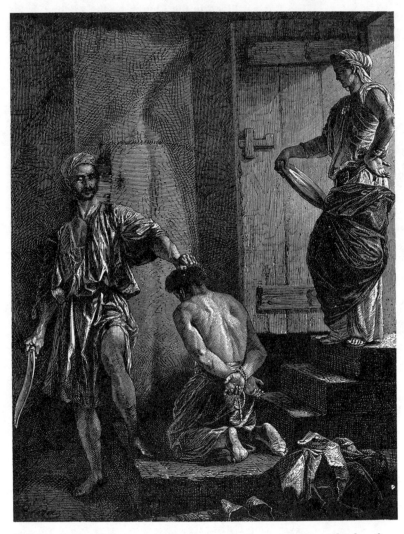

Salome, with silver tray in hand, awaits the execution of John the Baptist, so she could present his head to her mother, Queen Herodias.

was to be seven days of revelry, held in the courtyard of the palace garden.

Decorations of multi-colored ribbons were tied to silver rings which were imbedded in marble pillars. Gold and silver benches stood on pavements of black, red, white, and yellow marble. Drinks were served in golden goblets of many designs.

On the final day, when the king was half-drunk with wine, he told his seven eunichs:

> to bring Queen Vashti before the king
> with her royal crown in order to dis-
> play her beauty to the people and the
> princes, for she was beautiful.
> (Esther 1:11)

Queen Vashti refused. And this banquet of vain display by the king opened the way for Esther to save her people. And for Ahasuerus . . . his reign came to an abrupt halt in 465 B.C. when he was assassinated in bed.

**The Feast
where Salome
Danced**

When John the Baptist criticized the morals of Herodias, the bride of Herod, Herod had John locked in prison. Herod had divorced his first wife, a Nabatean princess, to marry Herodias who had been previously married to his own half-brother.

Herodias hated John the Baptist bitterly and looked for an opportunity to quickly dispatch him. Her chance finally came. It was Herod's birthday and he was giving a stag party for his palace aides, army officers and the leading citizens of Galilee.

And when the daughter of Herodias herself came in and danced, she pleased Herod and his dinner guests; and the king said to the girl [Salome], "Ask me for whatever you want and I will give it to you . . . whatever you ask of me, I will give it to you; up to half of my kingdom."

(Mark 6:22-23)

One can imagine what kind of dance Salome performed if it wielded enough influence to secure half of Herod's kingdom.

But Salome's mother, Herodias had other ideas. She told her daughter to ask for the head of John the Baptist on a platter.

Her wish was carried out!

Proper Occasions for Feasting

While worldly occasions for feasting are usually ones in which idolatry, drunkenness, vain display and immorality abound . . . there are times when, for the Christian, feasting is proper.

Sensible feasting is for

Refreshment (Lot and the two angels)
(Genesis 19:1-3)

Reconciliation (Laban makes peace with his family)
(Genesis 31:54,55)

Reunion (Joseph feasts his brethren)
(Genesis 43:16-34)

Restoration (Return of the prodigal son)
(Luke 15:22-24)

Perhaps every church should have a Feast of Reconciliation once a year where every member sits with those people he does not like. You recall the animosity that built up between Jacob and his father-in-law, Laban. Jacob was concerned because of Laban's cool attitude toward him. Laban accused him of stealing. And Jacob replied:

These 20 years I have been with you;
your ewes and your female goats have
not miscarried, nor have I eaten the
rams of your flocks . . .
. . . by day the heat consumed me,
and the frost by night,
and my sleep fled from my eyes.
These 20 years I have been in your house;
I served you fourteen years
for your two daughters,
and six years for your flock,
and you changed my wages ten times.
(Genesis 31:38-41)

Jacob had plenty of reason to be angry at Laban. But instead they made a monument of stones and it was called the Watchtower (Mizpah) . . . as a witness to their peace agreement.

Then Jacob presented a sacrifice to God and invited Laban and all his companions to a feast of reconciliation.

A Warning to World Leaders

I am rather amused when the President of the United States goes on a vacation and we see photos of him skiing or playing golf and the press releases that ensue tell of a "working" vacation.

Or when the President is toasting a Russian leader at a sumptuous banquet in Moscow and it is labeled a "working" banquet.

Scriptures warn us in Psalm 141 the danger of feasting with those who are God-denying:

Set a guard, O Lord, over my mouth;
Keep watch over the door of my lips.
Do not incline my heart to any evil thing,
To practice deeds of wickedness
With men who do iniquity;
And do not let me eat of their delicacies.
                    (Psalm 141:3-4)

How many free nations were sacrificed in the interest of détente at a "working" dinner!

We may not be eating wings of ostriches or the tongues of flamingoes today but Americans are still gorging themselves in feasts dripping with sickening sweets and laden with heart-degenerating fats and slaking it down with all kinds of liquors, whether it be Four Roses or Three Daffodils.

But these evils have one compensating factor.

They keep the doctors in business!

3

MUNCHIES, CRUNCHIES and FRENCH FRIES

**Don't
Steam
The
Roll**

Occasionally, when by necessity, I have to eat at a fast-food outlet (and you know their names), I throw the girl into a tizzy.

I order a hamburger and ask the girl not to steam or butter the roll. She looks at me quizzically as though I am unpatriotic.

Then I explain to her what I mean:

> Simply take the roll out of the box
> and do NOTHING with it
> . . . except put the hamburger on it.

To which she will question:

> You mean you don't want it steamed?
> It's so hard!

To which I reply:

> Exactly.
> Don't steam it.
> Don't butter it.
> Don't step on it.

By this time a long line has developed behind me and I'm looked at as "some kind of health nut."

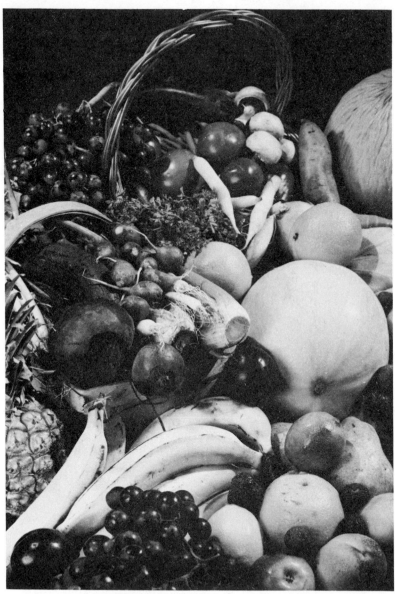

If you want to eat some wholesome foods, free of additives, you will have to go back to home gardening. Not only will the exercise be good for you in relieving the tensions of the day . . . but the resultant harvest will provide a physical bonus for your body!

An Average American Diet?

And nine times out of ten, when we get to the table, I throw the roll away anyway and just eat the hamburger . . . which ends up being between 18-20% fat!

For some, the typical American diet routine, particularly for youngsters, is rising in the morning dragged out . . . exclaiming:

> *Man, am I beat!*
> *Must of been that parsley I ate*
> *last night!*

To combat the fatigue we down a cola drink on the way to school, and become confused when our teacher shows us on the blackboard that 8 plus 8 does equal sixteen.

> *Wow, what a drag!*
> *I'm not a mathematical genius.*

The next big event for the student is protesting to make sure that "square" school principal designates "smoking rooms" for the students.

And to back up the dear students, their dear parents write irate letters and make irate phone calls demanding that the right of smoking not be denied.

> *After all, if we can eat butylated hydroxyanisole, parahydroxybenzoates and calcium propionate any time we want to, my son should be allowed to smoke!*
> What are you . . . some kind of discipline nut or something? Do you want my son to have a nervous breakdown!

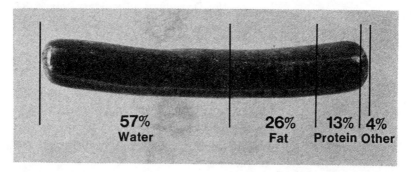

57%
Water

26%
Fat

13%
Protein

4%
Other

The good old American hot dog. Ralph Nader calls them *"among America's deadliest missiles."* Bess Myerson, former Consumer Affairs Commissioner of New York City said: *"After I found what was in hot dogs, I stopped eating them."*

According to the Department of Agriculture the average "all meat" hot dog contains 57% water, 26% fat, 13% protein and 2% corn syrup. The remainder includes salt, spices and various additives such as sodium erythorbate and sodium nitrite. And even kosher hot dogs contain these harmful additives!

**The
All-American
Lunch**

Well, now it's time for lunch. So we head for the nearest fast-food fare outlet and gorge ourselves with hamburgers and french fries. Where else but here can we "have it our way?"

Hamburgers . . . 18-20% fat.

French Fries . . . As American as your friendly undertaker!

Wherever possible, fried foods should be avoided . . . and particularly french fries. For in the frying process the composition of the oil is changed making it almost impossible for the fats to be assimilated into your blood stream. As a result they form into plaques on your arterial walls and are considered one of the major causes of heart attacks and strokes.

Well, now that you've had a wholesome breakfast and lunch interspersed with the necessary smoke break . . . it's time for a snack.

After all, old man fatigue is creeping in . . . and you need a pepper-upper. So you down a Mr. Goodbar. That makes you thirsty so you keep it company with a custard and a cola.

**The Sickly
Supper**

Now it's time for supper. Isn't it great to be alive! But first stop at the bakery and pick up one of those scrumptious oozy Angel Lee's Super-Fudge cake. After all . . . what's dinner without a dessert!

The All-American dinner . . . canned soup, frozen pizza, a cola drink and cake.

Must gulp it down in a hurry so I don't miss

my TV shows. I think I'd positively die if I missed As The World Turns. Man, do they have problems.

Funny, I'm hungry again. During the commercial I'll get some munchies and crunchies. They're so good I just can't stop eating them. Man that salt is tasty!

At midnight . . . our "well-fed," "nearly-dead" American wakes up . . . his stomach and his head doing flip-flops. But he has the answer. Quick, rush to the bathroom and down 2 pills for the tummy . . . that special kind that has simethecone!

As he nestles back into his bed he is heard to murmur . . .

> Knew I shouldn't have eaten
> that parsley.
> Man, that stuff could kill you!

Seem humorous?

How much of it is true in your own life?

Could this sketch be a partial reflection of a typical American daily diet?

Seduction by TV

Much of today's advertising uses what is termed subliminal seduction; that is, employing stimuli that exist or operate below the threshold of consciousness.

As an example, examine most cigarette advertising. It's true audibly they are selling you on the smooth taste, its "healthful" qualities of low tar . . . but all this is pictured in a setting of nature's outdoors . . . a refreshing stream, a wide prairie.

Or take a whiskey . . . the bottle does not dominate the ad or commercial. Instead you may see a man arriving at a mansion with a beautiful girl on his arm, alighting from his brand new Cadillac.

This subliminal seduction creates a picture in your mind of

cigarette - pure nature
whiskey   - success, prestige

Advertisers realize that the mind is quicker than the eye.

And if they can implant this idea of pure nature or success in your mind . . . you're already on the path to buying the product they are promoting!

$250,000 For One Minute!

The **preparation of** one minute commercials can run from $50,000 to as high as $250,000. Television commercials are the most carefully produced material in the entire field of mass communication.

Then **to buy** this one minute of time, advertisers must then spend an additional $25,000 to $250,000 or more per minute!

Sold on TV or through the print media by way of clever advertising . . . you really believe that "enriched food" is honestly better for you, that the good old American hot dog can do no harm even with its nitrates and nitrites, that candy will give you that burst of energy when you need it most, that puffed snacks will satisfy your hunger pangs.

In light of this brain-washing it is only natural for you to look down your nose at "health food fanatics."

Your criteria of thinking may be:

*If the Government ok'd it . . .
it's good enough for me.*

But what you fail to realize is that Government is made up of people engulfed in a hopeless tangle of beaurocracy . . . and they could be wrong. Even your doctor could be in error on vitamins and proper nutrition!

Because you eat these hollow calorie junk foods is all the more reason why you should consider 24-hour fasts at regular intervals.

Want some advice that is good for your health . . . and your budget? Here it is:

*When you shop,
pass by foods that are labeled
enriched or fortified.*

**Take
White Bread**

You will find these foods overpriced with very little of their original nutritional value left in them.

One nutritionist said white bread had one good benefit. It was good for picking up broken glass!

Enriched white bread costs 50 to 60 cents a pound. It is made from bleached white flour. With most of the original grain nutrients missing, about the only thing enriched about it are the pockets of the bread manufacturers.

Dr. Henry A. Schroeder of the Dartmouth Medical School testified at Senate hearings in the summer of 1970 that the milling process removes the following percentages of minerals which he describes as "essential for life or health."

Lost in the milling process:
40% of the chromium
86% of the manganese
89% of the cobalt
68% of the copper
78% of the zinc
48% of the molybdenium

None of these are replaced by "fortification" or "enrichment."

But you do get the undesirable chemical ingredients and preservatives.

You can make your own whole-wheat bread for just 47¢ worth of ingredients and you will end up with two pounds of bread!

Take Breakfast Cereals

If Jack Armstrong, "the all-American boy" subsisted on the dry breakfast cereals of today . . . he would be beset with health problems.

Most of the dry cereals have been so processed they lack potassium, which is vitally important to the health of your heart. Instead most are loaded with salt, BHT and BHA. A high salt (sodium-chloride) intake can lead to high blood pressure which leads to further complications including heart failure, strokes, and chronic kidney disease.

Synthetic Vitamins . . . a Bait

Many processors of foods used the adding of synthetic vitamins as a bait to the unwary consumer hoping that he will ignore the sugar, the saturated fats, the salt and chemicals that load up his product.

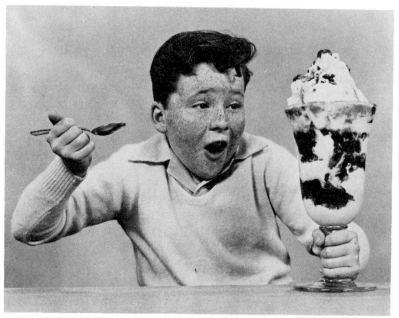

What this youngster is looking at is a pleasure for the palate but a nutritional disaster! This sundae is loaded with about 700 calories and 300 mg of sodium as well as a host of additives. How many times have you seen an obese person devouring a plate of ice cream? This sundae also abounds in the carbohydrate called sugar. Americans are over-sugared! U.S. bakeries prepare the equivalent of 50 million one-pound loaves of white bread a **day** and use nearly 3 million pounds of sugar in the process!

Sugar is the contributory cause of many illnesses. You would do well to consider it a poison to your body! How many times have you felt sluggish and headachy after an overindulgence in ice cream, chocolate cake or pie? Remember, the things that taste best are not always the best for you. Your indiscretions now will keep your doctor busy tomorrow! Fasting gives your body the opportunity to rid itself of poisons accumulated through bad eating habits.

Food Engineering, a magazine that reaches the food industry, estimates that to fortify any portion-size package of a food with 100% of the Recommended Adult Dietary Allowance of 9 vitamins costs less than one-fifth of a cent! Thus, it costs the manufacturer little . . . it increases sales . . . and you end up paying a higher cost for "enriched" foods that give you less nutrition!

Synthetic vitamins . . . those used in most "enriched" or "fortified" foods . . . are NOT the same as natural vitamins. Studies have shown that synthetic vitamins do not perform all the same functions of their natural components!

Ice Cream Isn't Nice Cream!

Are you old enough to remember the good old days of the handcrank freezer, filled with real cream, extra nonfat milk for higher protein, nuts, fruit, and genuine vanilla?

Those days are gone forever.

Now, when you buy ice cream it will most likely include:

plastic cream
    (known as concentrated milk fat)

dextrose	lactose
fructose	calcium hydroxide
cheese whey	sodium alginate
polysorbate 65	propylene glycol
gum acacia	
carboxymethylcellulose	

No wonder your body and particularly your digestive system needs a rest occasionally!

**Foods
I Avoid**

First, I've learned to not use salt. We get so easily into the habit of automatically picking up a salt shaker to season our meat, soup or vegetables. Foods have their own natural salt. You may believe that foods will taste flat without it. But I have learned, as have others, that foods take on a better taste without salt as your palate is freed from this chemical poison.

Those who already have heart disease, hardening of the arteries, high blood pressure and diseases of the kidneys, should definitely avoid the use of table salt.

As much as possible, I avoid all fried foods.

And, when given a choice, choose chicken over roast beef or steak.

Rarely do I eat any dessert. And instead of sugar in my herb tea, I use raw honey.

And as I write this book . . . what do I eat as a snack?

RAW, unsalted, ALMONDS. Almonds are high in mineral content and aid in preventing fatigue.

Well, this chapter is finished. Guess I'll go out to my garden and pick some parsley!

4

HOW'S YOUR LIVER, LATELY?

The scene was the United States Senate.
The hearings being held were on "Chemicals and the Future of Man."
The speaker, Senator Abraham Ribicoff.

> *Americans are becoming a nation of processed, packaged, and preserved people.*
>
> *We spend more than $60 billion for convenience foods including such items as TV dinners, snack foods of all kinds, and frozen foods.*
>
> *With these foods we consume every year more than 4 pounds of chemical preservatives, stabilizers, colorings, flavorings and other additives.*

Those remarks were made in April, 1971. Since then the figures have increased even more. In 1971 Americans were consuming more than 4 pounds of chemical preservatives, etc., Now, can you see why periodic fasts are recommended . . . to flush these poisons out of our system.

It is easy to understand how Americans are plagued with illness.

The sad fact is that the use of additives has doubled in the past 15 years, from 400 million pounds to more than 800 million pounds.

Today, over 3000 chemicals are deliberately added to our foods. Of course the food lobbyists will try to convince Americans that these chemicals are not harmful but rather enhance the food that we eat.

But chemicals and additives used in the raising and processing of food do contribute to the onset of disease. Most of these foreign substances do not add anything of nutritional value to the food (except greater profits for the producer). And they are irritating and often toxic to the bodily tissues.

**Your Life
Is In
Your Liver!**

Americans ingest these chemicals and additives seemingly without any ill effect. For this they can thank their liver, and other detoxifying and eliminating organs that are able either to neutralize or dispose of them.

The liver is the largest and perhaps the most complicated organ in the body. It is the key unit in the processing of food nutrients, and acts as a filter, neutralizing waste products.

When the liver malfunctions it is oftentimes blamed on the gall bladder. In one survey of the Mayo Clinic, it found that 56% of all their patients who had their gall bladder removed had their original troubles return in full violence:

belching
heartburn
flatulence
constipation
intolerance to fats
an uncomfortable sense of
  fullness after eating

Chemicals and food additives may cause liver poisoning particularly in their accumulated use over the years. Extreme fatigue, loss of appetite and a general sluggish feeling may indicate that the liver is failing. Your doctor is able to perform liver-function tests with your blood and urine to determine accurately the adequacy or inadequacy of your liver function.

While we can live without a gall bladder and some other organs, it is not possible to live without a liver.

The liver is by far, the most versatile of all organs of the body, so indispensable that without it the body would perish in 24 hours.

And through this most valuable organ . . . without which we cannot live . . . must pass the over 3000 chemicals and additives which we may ingest.

In other words, we make the liver the whipping boy for our indiscretion in eating.

Before the days of additives and chemicals the liver had a full time job as the filter of the body, removing or neutralizing waste products. Now we have complicated and overburdened its functions with a myriad number of chemical preservatives. Is it any wonder we are plagued with commercials on antacids that promise glorious things for our tummy?

And Demanding Consumers Don't Help

One medical textbook begins its chapter on Additives and Pesticides in Foods as follows:

> The complexities of modern urbanized society have placed increasing demands on growers and processors of food for products of uniform composition with organoleptic appeal, of good keeping quality, in sanitary, packaged form, and convenient to prepare in the home.[1]

Many doctors and medical textbooks like to use big words. Somehow they have an official ring to them, that no laymen would dare challenge, and tends to place them in a holy circle of knowledge that is beyond question.

Now what in the world does "organoleptic appeal" mean? And could not a more common word or phrase be used to convey the thought? Yes! Organoleptic appeal means that the processor of foods wants to produce a product that will appeal to the senses of the buyer . . . such as the senses of taste, smell, and touch.

Now the writer's opening paragraph is certainly honest. It is also revealing. It shows that to some degree, you and I as consum-

---

[1]Goodhart and Shils: Modern Nutrition in Health and Disease, (Philadelphia: Lea & Febiger), 1973, p. 434.

ers are to blame for the chemicals and additives that have been added to our foods.

With the population explosion . . . the greater demands for food at lowest prices . . . we are willing (or most people are) to sacrifice wholesomeness and a little inconvenience, for food that is uniform in composition . . . is appealing to our senses and to our eyes and is uniform in quality and above all . . . plastic wrapped!

Functions of Food Additives

What are the functions of food additives? There are 9 basic areas where food additives are used:

1. Acids, Alkalies and Buffering Agents

Used primarily in the dairy, brewing and baking industries to neutralize acid foods and also to impart the acidity which is characteristic of foods such as soft drinks and confections.

Examples:
phosphoric, malic and fumaric acids, glucono-delta-lactone, sodium, calcium and magnesium hydroxides.

2. Preservatives

Used to inhibit or prevent spoilage due to yeasts, molds or bacteria.

Examples:
benzoic acid, methyl and propyl parahydroxybenzoates, sulfur dioxide, sodium and calcium propionate.

3. Antioxidants

Added to retard rancidity and other changes of an oxidative nature in vegetable or animal oils and fats.

Examples:
butylated hydroxyanisole (BHA), butylhydroxytoluene (BHT).

4. Emulsifying agents

Used to effect a dispersion of oils in a watery media and vice versa. Used widely in margarine, salad dressings, cheese spreads and candy, as well as in the baking industry.

Examples:

mono and di-glycerides, polyoxyethylene and sorbitan esters.

5. Sequestrants

Used to bind (or chelate) trace metals which may change flavor or color in certain products.

Example:

ethylene-diamine tetraacetic acid (EDTA).

6. Flavoring Agents

Used not only to add an aromatic property to food but also to mask objectional qualities of the food that may deter the consumer from buying.

Examples:

eugenol, diacetal, cinnamic aldehyde, methyl anthranilate, methyl salicylate.

7. Stabilizers

Used to impart texture and body to foods such as processed cheese, soups and candies.

Examples:

Alginates, carrageen, synthetic cellulosic gums.

8. Bleaching Agents

These are used by the baking industry chiefly to quicken the oxidation of flour.

Examples:

Benzoyl peroxide, chlorine dioxide, potassium bromate, acetone peroxide, azo-dicarbonamide.

9. **Texturizing Agents**
   These are used to make sure pickles and canned vegetables remain firm and crisp.
   Examples:
   Alums such as potassium or sodium aluminum sulfate.

Now, you might ask the question . . . what in the world does all this have to do with fasting? Everything.

No Wonder We Get Sick

With all these additives pumped into our foods (and we have not even fully covered the subject) . . . is it no wonder that our digestive system needs a rest so the poisons can be periodically flushed out!

We're not finished yet, either!

The Curse of Indirect Additives (or MORE POISONS AT NO ADDED COST)

Everything seems to come packaged these days . . . from our hamburgers to our ham hocks!

The largest single group of indirect additives are made up of the components of food packaging materials. The foods rub against the inside of the box and we digest a bit of whatever was sprayed upon it!

Waxes and synthetic polymeric resins are used to coat paperboard packaging materials. Resins and lacquers are found on metallic containers.

Then there is a multitude of chemical components used to make sure a container is either stable or flexible, grease resistant or moisture repellant.

Chemicals used also in processing food prior to packaging can finally filter down to our liver. Defoaming and wetting agents

The Evening Bulletin

WEDNESDAY, AUGUST 20, 1975   BB

Filth in Baby Food Reported

Bulletin Wire Services

Washington — Tests on major brands of baby food showed small amounts of insects, insect parts and rodent hairs present in about one-quart the samples, Con-

sumers Union reports.

CU also said yesterday it found paint chips in some of the foods from enamel which flaked off the inside of the lid.

Although it said it did not regard

The FDA said it has no specific tolerance level for filth in baby food but does for some of the products which might go into it, such as fruit and cereals. Small amounts of some contaminants are regarded by the

'Antsy' kids
Food additives called hyperactivity's cause

WASHINGTON (P) — About half the nation's hyperactive children, whose erratic behavior often makes them miserable failures in school, could be successfully treated simply by removing artificial flavors and colors from their food,

the hyperactive children began following an additive-free diet.

Feingold, who said he has successfully treated, hundreds of hyperactive children, said the disorder has reached "epidemic proportions" and now may afflict more than f...

tioned that the syndrome has various symptoms and may have many causes — psychosocial, environmental and nutritional.

A federal interagency task force is setting up a study to prove or disprove Feingold's theory scien-

Food Coloring Is Under the Gun
FDA Hunts Link to Childhood Malady

By KATHY HACKER
Bulletin Food Editor

TWO YEARGS AGO, a California allergist caused a national stir by proposing a direct link between hyperactivity among children and the consumption of artificial colorings and flavorings ro... cessed

Aft... manen, Benjar sters that a States aggre be r chem, Si gered ers, food flavo ucts N steps bu: f

hert C. Kolbye Jr., associate director for sciences with the Bureau of Foods, the FDA is organizing, a federal work group to "jointly fund and design the protocols needed to either prove or disprove Dr. Feingold's theories," according to a memo from a meeting between Feingold and FDA Commissioner Alexander ... the memo ...

orings in the ingredient listings. At present, Feingold's diet is difficult—if not impossible— to follow since a great percentage of packaged foods contain the suspect additives and often are not clearly labeled. Feingold claims that, when even a small quantity of artificial additive is consumed, symptoms of hyperkinesis ... chi...

Five Ill From Canned Juice Containing Tin, FDA Says

WASHINGTON (P) — Five persons became ill after drinking Campbell V-8 Cocktail Vegetable Juice containing high levels of tin, the Food and Drug Administration said Thursday.

After being notified of the

3 3-C U-5V   ZCN and 33-CU-5V5ZDN.

Asked why announcement of the recall was delayed for six weeks, the FDA said it had to await a report from its laboratories on the level of tin in the

These newspaper headlines, gathered from just one week's news are indicative of the problems we face in the foods we eat.

and fumigants are typical examples.

Foods derived from livestock and poultry contain indirect additives that we gobble up as consumers. Poultry feed contains growth promoting agents such as coccidiostats, antibiotics and organic arsenicals. Stilbestrol, a hormone used to force the growth of cattle and poultry, becomes an indirect additive which one day may be revealed as a major factor in disrupting bodily functions.

There are numerous controversies both among scientists and regulatory agencies surrounding the use of food additives.

But common sense dictates to me that the more natural the source of the food . . . the less tampered with . . . the more wholesome and nutritious it will be.

But because of today's living and the almost impossibility of securing food that has not been loaded with propyl parahydroxybenzoates, BHA, BHT, ethylenediamine tetraacetic acid, methyl anthranilate, aluminum sulfate and a multitude of other chemical components . . . I find my reasons for fasting even more of a vital necessity!

I find it amazing how brain-washed most Americans are on what constitutes good nutrition . . . and I include some doctors in this category, too. Many physicians feel if you eat proper meals you will have an adequate diet . . . adequate for what . . . becoming a hospital patient?

Conversation of Tomorrow

Imagine walking down the street and meeting a friend and this conversation taking place.

Hi! Bill,
Just came from lunch!
What did you have?
I had glucono-delta-lactone and calcium propionate with butylhydroxytoluene topped off with parsley. But I got a miserable headache. Must of been the parsley. I knew I shouldn't have eaten it.
You're right, Tom.
That parsley will do it every time! You're not supposed to eat that stuff. It's just window dressing. Man . . . that could kill you!

The "Miracle" Additives

Benzoic acid, a chemical preservative, found in fruit juices, pickles, preserves and in soft drinks, is a mild irritant to the skin, eyes and mucous membranes. The Soviet Union has restricted use of this chemical in their foods because tests indicated that it contributed to tension and stress.

Butylated hydroxyanisole (BHA), is perhaps the most widely used antioxidant in use in the United States today. It is used in ice cream, in candy, baked goods, dry breakfast cereals, nuts, soup mixes, etc. Various experiments have been made with this chemical which indicated that BHA inhibits the contraction of smooth muscles of the intestine in the ileum area.

Butylated hydroxytoluene (BHT), a widely used antioxidant. It is used in chewing gum, dry breakfast cereals, freeze-dried meats and sometimes used in conjunction with BHA. BHT appears to be even more toxic than BHA. Adverse findings include metabolic stress, loss of weight, increase of liver weight, damage to liver and kidneys, increase of serum cholesterol and phospholipid levels and baldness. Some also believe it contributes to chronic, disabling asthmatic attacks, fatigue and difficulty in breathing.

Calcium propionate, a chemical preservative. You will find it used in bread, rolls and most baked goods. It is also used in chocolate products, in processes cheeses, in pizza crusts, etc. Often this chemical is combined with sodium propionate. It has been reported that these chemicals cause allergic reactions that begin 4-18 hours after eating foods with these additives.

These adverse reactions are similar to a gall-bladder attack and may end with a partial or total migraine headache.

Chinese Syndrome

Monosodium glutamate (MSG) is a so-called "flavor enhancer." It is widely used and hence hard to avoid in any processed food. It is found in the convenience "heat-and-serve" foods, in canned soups, in meats and meat tenderizers, in fish fillets, clam chowder, poultry, pickles, salad dressing, and candy.

Why is it used so extensively? Because it helps to maintain that fresh-cooked quality and supposedly restores flavor. House-

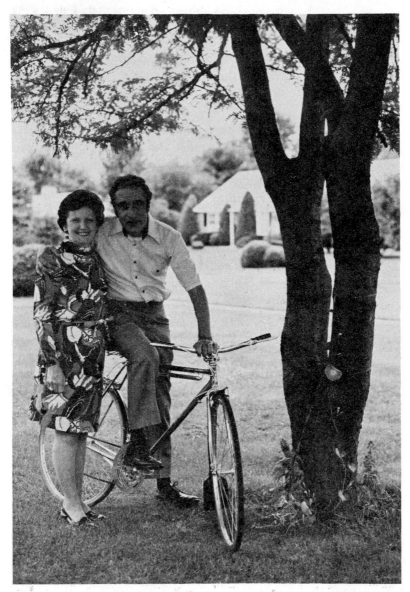

My dear wife, Mary, and I relax under a tree on a front yard. Note the morning glory growing up our sunburst locust. Next to parsley, morning glories are my favorite plant. By the way, bike riding is another form of mild, beneficial exercise.

wives are encouraged to sprinkle it on raw or cooked meats and vegetables.

Dr. Robert Ho Man Kowk in writing in The New England Journal of Medicine (1968) reported a strange syndrome which later was called the "Chinese syndrome." After eating in a Chinese restaurant he developed "numbness at the back of the neck, gradually radiating to both arms and the back, general weakness and palpitations." In animal experimentation with MSG (monosodium glutamate) brain lesions occurred. Baby food manufacturers decided to discontinue the use of MSG because of adverse findings.

It is not the purpose of this book to provide a long medical dissertation on chemical additives with pages of bibliography. Anyone who wishes to find further information will find such readily available both in medical and nutritional books and reports.

The layman is not interested in all the technicalities. His greatest concern is: "Is the food I eat wholesome and nutritious for my children and for my own body?"

In all honesty, after reading many reports, my own personal conclusion is that commercial, processed food, for the most part cannot meet this requirement.

The more an individual can rely on the food produced in his own backyard garden . . . the better chance he stands for a longer life.

**Show Me
Your Liver
and I'll Show You
Your Life!**

In Ezekiel 21:21, when the king of Babylon had to decide which of two routes he should take ... whether to attack Jerusalem or Rabbah (in Jordan)

> he shakes the arrows,
> he consults the household idols,
> he looks at the liver.

The liver has four lobes, five ligaments, five fissures, and five sets of vessels. To slaughter an animal and examine the liver was a very common type of divination by which those in ancient days who knew not the one true God thought they could obtain information about the future.

Every year you pour into your body some 4 pounds of chemicals in the form of preservatives, stabilizers and additives that must pass through a 3-4 pound liver through cells clustered in groups called lobules (each lobule about 1/25 inch in diameter) so these impurities can be filtered and neutralized.

Kings-of-old slaughtered animals to inspect their livers and find out which way to turn. If a doctor could examine your liver today, he would know much about your future life or your lack of a future!

By the way, how's your liver, lately?

5

DANIEL HAD A BETTER WAY

The Bible reminds us:

*. . . do you not know that your body
is a temple of the Holy Spirit
who is in you,
whom ye have from God,
and that ye are not your own?
For you have been bought with a price:
therefore glorify God in your body.*
                    (1 Corinthians 6:19-20)

Now, how can you glorify your body by dumping

polysorbate 65
sodium alginate
polyoxyethylene
calcium propionate

and a host of other chemicals into it daily?

Some people treat their car better than they take care of their body!

Daniel's Diet Gave Him 2 Kingdoms

About 606 B.C., after Babylon's King Nebuchadnezzar had conquered Jerusalem, he ordered his aide to select young men of the royal family and nobility of Judah to teach them the Chaldean language and literature.

The aide was instructed by Nebuchadnezzar to pick strong, healthy lads.

The aide came back with many young men, among whom were Daniel and three of his friends. They were quickly given Babylonian names.

Daniel was called Belteshazzar
Hananiah was called Shadrach
Misha-el was called Meshach
Azariah was called Abednego

The king assigned them the best of food and wine from his own kitchen during this three-year training period. His plan was to appoint them to governmental offices when they graduated.

**Daniel
Refused
The King's Food**

Daniel and his friends, however, did not want to eat the food and wine prescribed by the king.

This alarmed the commander who said:

I am afraid of my lord the king, who has appointed your food and your drink; for why should he see your faces looking more haggard than the youths who are your own age? Then you would make me forfeit my head to the king.

(Daniel 1:10)

Daniel talked it over with the steward and finally suggested a 10-day test.

Here was the test:

Daniel and his 3 friends would eat only vegetables and water for 10 days.

The other young men would eat the king's rich diet which included meat and wine.

The steward agreed to the test.

The Vegetable Diet

Most likely the vegetables that Daniel ate included grains, lentils and basic vegetables.

You see, Daniel had:

> ... made up his mind that he would not defile himself with the king's choice food or with the wine which he drank ...
>
> *(Daniel 1:8)*

Why did they not want to eat the "king's choice food"?

There were two basic reasons:

1. The food would include meat declared unclean by the law of Moses (See Leviticus 11 or Deuteronomy 14:3-20).

2. It would regularly be food which had been first offered to the Babylonian gods.

And perhaps there was also a lingering third reason:

3. Daniel and his friends may have also looked upon the Babylonian fancy diet as unhealthy.

Imagine . . . Daniel and his friends, coming from a captured land . . . right into favor with the King of Babylon.

Here they were offered the best of food the King had to offer, meat and wine.

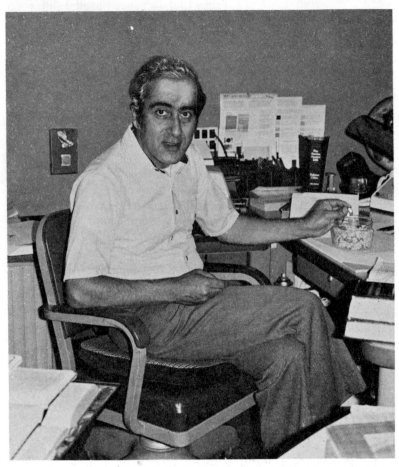

Don't nibble on munchies, crunchies and french fries when you are
hungry. These are hollow junk foods loaded with poisonous additives
that contribute to making you nervous, irritable and fatigued. I always
keep a jar of raw, **unsalted** mixed nuts next to me ... almonds,
sunflower seeds and soybeans. And for an extra thrill, throw in unsul-
phered raisins!

And they turned it down for vegetables and water!

One can imagine how the other students laughed at them. Perhaps they were the first "health nuts" to bear the ridicule of friends.

But even today . . . let someone tell a friend he is fasting . . . or let him omit from his regular diet coffee, colas and desserts in favor of bean sprouts and water and he will be looked on as some kind of oddball.

Daniel Had a Better Idea!

Advertisers in the fast-food industry bombard us on TV with clowns jumping around with hamburgers and french fries. And it would seem totally un-American not to patronize them.

But Daniel had a better idea!

His desire was to serve and honor God. He realized his body belonged to God and was to kept holy. And he and his companions did not want anything to enter their body that would defile it and be dishonoring to the God whom they loved and whom they served.

So the 10-day test began.

Can you picture the scene in the dining room?

Waiters come in where about 50 or 60 young men are seated. Piled high on trays are succulent portions of meat . . . their aroma wafting over the tables. They place the steaming trays down at each table along with a rich, red wine . . . that is, at every table except Daniel's.

The other youths plunge into their full course dinner, inwardly thankful they did not choose the course that Daniel selected. As they gobble their meat, their eyes turn toward Daniel's table.

And what do they see?

UGH!

What a concoction! How could anyone possibly exist on that junk? Why, they would be famished within the hour! They would starve!

The waiter comes to Daniel's table . . . he sets down a tray of what, to many, would appear to be unappetizing vegetables and a pitcher of water. Who knows . . . perhaps a conglomerate of bean and alfalfa or lentil sprouts and herbs.

Do you think the youths at the meat tables may have turned in scorn at Daniel and sang in chorus:

Have it your way . . .
HAVE IT your way!

Well, Daniel did have it his way . . . to the very last bean sprout!

The Results of the 10-day Test

And what happened?

The Bible tells us the result of this 10-day test.

> At the end of ten days their appearance [Daniel's and his 3 companions] seemed better and they were fatter than all the youths who had been eating the king's choice food.
> So the overseer continued to withhold their choice food and the wine they

*were to drink, and kept giving them
vegetables.*

(Daniel 1:15-16)

How did God bless them when they followed His leading in sensible eating and
being uncompromising with worldly
standards?

*As for the four youths, God gave them
knowledge and intelligence in every
branch of literature and wisdom;
Daniel even understood all kinds of
visions and dreams.*

(Daniel 1:17)

**Nebuchadnezzar's
Reaction**

And what was King Nebuchadnezzar's reaction at the end of their training period?

*And the king talked with them,
and out of them all
not one was found like
Daniel, Hananiah, Mishael
and Azariah;
so they entered the king's
personal service.*

(Daniel 1:19)

And what did Nebuchadnezzar discover in
the quality of their living?

*And as for every matter
of wisdom and understanding
about which the king consulted them,
he found them ten times better
than all the magicians and conjurers
who were in all his realm.*

(Daniel 1:20)

Now, wait a minute!

Before you discount the entire story . . .
think about it for a minute.

It makes sense! Good common sense.

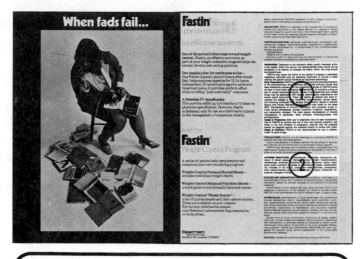

The above ad appeared in *Emergency Medicine*, September, 1975. It recommends a drug for weight control called **FASTIN.** Note the adverse reactions. Dr. Allan Cott, a psychiatrist at Gracie Square Hospital in New York City reports: *"From my observations, I'd say that the chances are much better for permanent weight control after fasting than after any other diet."*

Dr. Siegfried Heyden, professor of community health sciences at Duke University, agrees. He remarks: *"Spectacular weight losses have been recorded by fasting. And fasts up to two days are perfectly safe even without the supervision of a doctor. Fasts for longer periods might be equally as safe, but should be done under medical supervision."*

Daniel's Wisdom Should Be Ours

In this three-year training period . . . Daniel and his companions made sure that any food that entered their body was wholesome and beneficial. For ten days they ate nothing but vegetables and water. This does not imply that they continued this diet the entire three years without eating any meat; although this could be possible.

They certainly did not eat or drink anything that was unclean or offered first to idols; nor did they drink the strong Babylonian wines with their unclean additives.

Because of their sensible eating habits:

1. They were better physically
2. They were better mentally
3. They were stronger spiritually

Even the godless King Nebuchadnezzar recognized this fact.

Daniel, in fact — by a special gift of God — even understood and could interpret dreams and visions. And he and his companions, as acknowledged by King Nebuchadnezzar were ten times better in their wisdom and understanding than all his other counsellors.

This is not to imply that if you go on this diet you will be able to interpret dreams and visions. However, if does mean that, even in our eating and drinking, if we honor God and our body (His Temple), God will honor us with blessings.

**Give Up
Those
Junk Foods
and Start Living!**

You might ask . . . well, what does this all lead to?

Practically, I mean . . . for me?

Well, you can't undo the damage you have done to your body over the years by eating junk foods, fried foods, fats, gooey desserts, sugars, salt . . . and every time you have a sniffle rushing to the doctor to load yourself up with drugs.

But you can clean out your system regularly by fasting to cleanse your system of existing impurities in your body . . . some which have lodged in your organs, perhaps for many, many years!

And while you continue this periodic cleansing in fasting you can also spend the meal times as of old in prayer!

Let me explain it this way.

Suppose someone gave you a brand new Cadillac. Then, suppose you put kerosene in the gas tank because a nearby truck-stop sold only kerosene. And you replaced the oil only with the cheapest grade non-detergent fluids.

Wouldn't that dishonor both the gift and the giver?

Then, too, the way you feed your body reflects either honor or dishonor to the Giver.

With this understanding you can determine to eat foods that honor your body instead of those which damage it.

It means — in my opinion — giving up among other things:

fast-food drive-in type restaurants that specialize in hamburgers, french fries, fried chicken and colas.

hot dogs
pickles
coffee and tea
    (Herb teas are fine, however)
sugar and salt
cold cuts that have nitrite
    and nitrate
all sugary desserts, pies
    and ice cream
TV dinners
smoking
drinking of alcoholic beverages

At this point, you may feel life is simply not worth living.

On the contrary, when you start substituting the junk you have been eating with wholesome foods . . . that's when you WILL START LIVING.

You won't wake up dragged out in the morning . . . fatigued in mid-afternoon and have a blinding headache at night, finding yourself unable to sleep. You won't find yourself being more at home in a doctor's waiting room than in your own living room.

Don't Expect a Miracle Overnight!

Now, after years of damaging your body . . . don't expect a 24-hour miracle on your first fast. You cannot undo in 24 hours what you have done in 20 or 40 years of unwise living.

But you will see your physical, mental and spiritual acuity sharpen. What is acuity? Acuity is sharpness, alertness, and clearness of perception in your being!

For once in your life . . . you'll feel ALIVE!

And because of this heightened acuity, you will be able at least partially to increase in wisdom and in understanding . . . just as Daniel and his three companions did.

And your appearance and overall physical well-being will improve.

Have you looked into your mirror lately?

Do you see wrinkles?

Are there bags under your eyes?

Are you getting paunchy?

Are you overweight? An optimist is a girl who mistakes a bulge for a curve.

Perhaps if you tried it "your way" for these many years . . . and feel dull, dragged out and depressed . . . you might take an example from the Bible and try Daniel's menu for better living.

After all, Daniel had a BETTER way!

6

YOU MEAN HIPPOCRATES FASTED?

Bowker's Medical Books in Print, 1975 edition, lists over 28,000 titles of medical books in 5000 subject categories available from some 1060 publishers.

Of the 28,000 medical books, only 4 books are listed under FASTING.

Hippocrates, often called the "father of medicine," probably would turn over in his grave if he knew this.

You mean Hippocrates fasted?

Well, I never met him personally . . . but I can tell you this, "I never saw him at MacDonalds!"

But I do recall him saying:

> Abstinence and quiet
> cure many diseases

And in Ecclesiasticus, the longest and one of the most important books of the Apocrypha, we are warned:

> He that sinneth before his Maker,
> let him fall
> into the hands of a physician.

And Benjamin Franklin reminds us:

*He's the best physician that knows
the worthlessness of most medicines.*

I am amazed that the American Medical Association has not seen to it that more books were written on fasting and its merits.

The over 1100 page book, Modern Nutrition in Health and Disease contains only 20 lines on fasting and these 20 lines are nega-

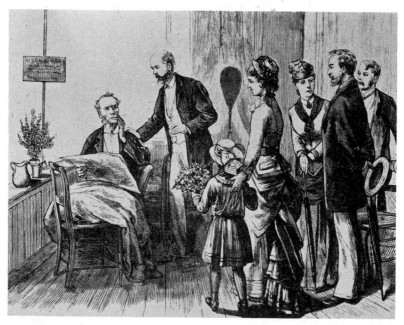

Dr. Tanner, a medical doctor, in the 1880's, went on a 40 day fast. This scene shows his doctor and anxious relatives visiting him. Fasting was considered an unusual event that brought newspaper coverage.

tive in their content. Yet this is a medical book found on most doctor's shelves!

Hippocrates was an outstanding physician in his time. Born about 460 B.C., he was the son of a physician and grew up and practiced among the thousands of invalids who came to the hot springs of Cos, an island off of Greece. Cos, later became a navigational point for Paul's ship on the voyage from Ephesus to Rhodes (Acts 21:1).

Diet Rather than Drugs

Now Hippocrates had a teacher named Herodicus. It was Herodicus who formed his art by teaching Hippocrates to rely upon diet and exercise rather than upon drugs.

Now this was not the 20th century A.D. This was the 5th Century B.C.! And that rule of good health is still valid (if not more valid with our pollutants) today!

And by pollutants, I mean not only the pollutants in the air we breathe and the food we eat but also in the medical drugs we ingest!

The success of Hippocrates was so widespread that the rulers of both Macedon (Northern Greece) and Persia were among his patients.

Hippocrates wrote textbooks for physicians . . . and clinical records that were not to be equalled for over 1700 years! He also set a high standard for medical honesty, admitting that in 60% of the cases, the disease, or the treatment, proved fatal.

**Nature . . .
The
Principal
Healer**

Hippocrates believed that nature was the principal healer . . . and that all the physician could do was to remove or reduce the impediments to this natural defense and recuperation. This is why Hippocrates made little use of drugs.

Fasting was often prescribed by Hippocrates. He believed:

*the more we nourish unhealthy bodies
the more we injure them.*

He also believed man should have only one meal a day.

It is interesting to note that in the Hippocratic treatise, On the Physician, he gave detailed directions for the preparation of the operating room, the arrangement of natural and artificial light, the cleanliness of the hands and the care and use of instruments, as well as the position of the patients and the bandaging of wounds.

And this was over 2400 years ago!

Even at that time, physicians were well paid and received as much as an equivalent of today's $12,000 a year. The average annual income today can vary from $35,000 to $48,000 plus almost free medical care!

It was Hippocrates who, because of his concern for high medical ethics, who, in part, was responsible for creating The Hippocratic Oath.

While medical graduates give it lip service today in their graduation ceremonies, I believe it wise to print it here. It will give you an idea how far many physicians have departed from a set of standards set down by the father of medicine.

The Hippocratic Oath

I swear by Apollo Physician, by Asclepius, by Hygiaea, by Panacea, and by all the gods and goddesses, making them my witnesses, that I will carry out, according to my ability and judgment, this oath and this indenture

(Asclepius was the Greek god of Medicine. Hygiaea was the goddess of Health. Panacea was the goddess of Healing.)

*To hold my teacher in this art
equal to my own parents;
to make him partner in my livelihood;
when he is in need of money
to share mine with him;
to consider his family as my own brothers,
and to teach them this art,
if they want to learn it,
without fee or indenture:*

(How many doctors today would go this far as to hold their teachers equal to their own parents, to share their money, when a need arises, and to teach this art of medicine to others, without cost?)

*to impart precept, oral instruction,
and all other instruction
to my own sons, to the sons of my teacher,
and to indentured pupils
who have taken the physician's oath,
but to no one else.
I will use treatment to help the sick
according to my ability and judgment,*

but never with a view to injury and
  wrongdoing.
Neither will I administer a poison to
  anybody when asked to do so,
nor will I suggest such a course.
Similarly I will not give to a woman a
  pessary to cause abortion.
But I will keep pure and holy
both my life and my art.

> (This part of the oath is certainly ignored
> today in our so-called 20th century en-
> lightened society where doctors perform
> thousands of abortions daily!)

I will not use the knife,
not even, verily, on sufferers from stone,
but I will give place to such as are
  craftsmen therein.

Into whatsoever houses I enter
I will enter to help the sick,
and I will abstain
from all intentional wrongdoing and
  harm.
especially from abusing the bodies
of man or woman, bond or free.
And whatsoever I shall see or hear
  in the course of my profession,
as well as outside my profession
in my communication with men,
if it be what should not be published abroad,
I will never divulge,
holding such things to be
holy secrets.

Now if I carry out this oath,
and break it not,
may I gain forever reputation among all
  men
for my life and for my art;
but if I transgress it
and forswear myself,
may the opposite befall me.

Hippocrates then also gives some good advice to physicians which included the following:

Sometimes give your services for nothing;
and if there be an opportunity of serving a
stranger
who is in financial straits,
give him full assistance.
For where there is love of man,
there is also love of art.

(We can be truly thankful for every one of today's physicians who is indeed a lover of his fellow man and who shows this by reasonable charges. We can only deplore that yacht club minority whose fees, sometimes for only the work of moments, break the financial backs of their helpless patients.)

Hippocrates died at the ripe, old age of 83, having left a great legacy for the medical profession to follow.

And many, in fact, perhaps the majority, in the medical profession do seek to uphold these ideals.

What is the Real Purpose of the American Medical Association?

It is sad that the American Medical Association which was founded to promote the science and art of medicine and the betterment of public health has mushroomed into a powerful lobbying group.

One report alleges that the American Medical Political Action Committee (AMPAC), from 1962-1974, collected more than $12 million from AMA member doctors and fed it into the campaign chests of legislators whose favor AMA lobbyists wished to nurture.

The Charlotte Observer

Foremost Newspaper Of The Carolinas

90th Year—No. 144   TUESDAY, SEPTEMBER 9, 1975   32 Pages   Price 15 Cents

MDs Charged High Fees
To Give Dangerous Drug

Dangerous Drug Nearly Given Okay

UNNECESSARY SURGERY

How much unnecessary surgery is performed in the United States each year? No one knows for sure.

In 1938 Dr. Richard Cabot, professor of medicine at Harvard, declared, "The greatest single curse in medicine is the curse of unnecessary operations, and there would be fewer of them, if the doctor got the same salary whether he operated or not."

FDA, Doctors Differ on Listing All Drug Effects

SHOULD THERE BE a federal requirement that all patients be told about all possible side effects of the medicines their doctors prescribe?

Yes, say federal drug officials.

No, say medical society representatives here and nationally.

The U.S. Food and Drug Administration (FDA) wants lists of side effects included with many prescription drugs.

Such lists, known as Patient Package Inserts (PPI), already accompany oral contraceptives and the prospects are that the practice will be extended to other drugs.

The Food and Drug Administration contends the side effects should be listed so patients will be alert to the possible symptoms and report them to their doctors sooner.

Unnecessary Surgery Costly, Panel Is Told

WASHINGTON—(AP)—In the winter of 1969, Mrs. Marie Valenzuela of Woodlawn, Calif., was told her daughter, who had a fever, needed her tonsils removed.

Before this doctor was finished, he had

the hospital suffering shock over the condition of her child.

The story was related Tuesday to a House Commerce investigations subcommittee

as many as 3.2 million surgical operations may be performed needlessly each year in the United States.

The cost to patients for unnecessary

Evening Bulletin   Thursday, August 21, 1975

Oral Diabetic Drugs Attacked as Perilous, Often Useless

These newspaper headlines reveal the danger of drugs and the excesses in unnecessary surgery.

Another disclosure document alleged instances of close AMA cooperation with the nation's $8 billion-a-year pharmaceutical industry.

**Famous
Fasters**

Socrates and Plato fasted periodically. And Pythagoras, a Greek philosopher, reportedly did a 40-day fast before he took his examination at the University in Alexandria.

His reason: it cleared his head. He asked his students to follow his example.

The Egyptians and the Druids fasted. So did the British suffragettes — "to publicize the inferior status of women."

In Russia, Tolstoy fasted. He marked:

> to refuse food and drink . . .
> is more than pleasure,
> it is the joy of the soul.

American Indians, the Puritans and Benjamin Franklin fasted, as well.

Fasting was very popular in the late 19th century but since then has almost faded into oblivion.

Many in the medical profession look skeptically at fasting as having any therapeutic benefit. The late Alice Chase wrote:

> The medical profession, ruling over the health of mankind, appears willing to subject the sick to the trial of all sorts of drugs, surgery, electric shock, and other forms of treatment that are experimental, even heroic — and sometimes useless.

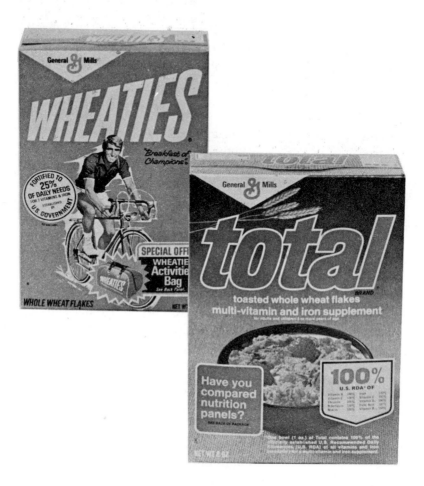

Jim Hightower, in his book, *Eat Your Heart Out: How Food Profiteers Victimize the Consumer,* lambasts the government and the food industry for promoting monopolistic practices that have made *"the price of food go up and the quality go down."*

While there are some 32,000 food manufacturing firms in America, just about 50 of these companies already make about three-quarters of the industry's profits.

Wheaties cost around 53 cents for a regular size box. Yet, he alleges, there is no more than two cents worth of wheat in Wheaties; the box costs more than that. Total is Wheaties plus a half-cent worth of vitamins sprayed on, but sold for 22 cents more!

They are unwilling to open their minds and eyes to the more kindly procedures such as rest of the body, mind and emotions.

And, of course, it is fasting that provides rest to the body, mind and emotions!

The Paradox of Hospitals

Dr. Allan Cott, in his book, FASTING: The Ultimate Diet, states:

If the medical profession were really "tuned in" to nutrition, would the waiting rooms of doctors' offices be "sweetened" with bowls of caramels and candy corn and jawbreakers and lollipops and all-day suckers?

Would the corridors and the recreation rooms of hospitals be lined with vending machines purveying chocolate bars, sugary and carbonated soft drinks, potato chips, and other junk foods containing preservatives, additives, artificial coloring – with practically no nutritional value?

Would cigarettes be on sale? Apples and carrot sticks and sunflower seeds and raw nuts and raisins and toasted soybeans – that will be the day you find them there![1]

Dr. Cott goes on to say:

The cliché "we are what we eat" no longer refers only to our physical being; it refers to our mental health as well. The state of nutrition affects our behavior and our mood, and can affect our sanity.[2]

---

[1]Alan Cott, M.D., Fasting: The Ultimate Diet (New York: Bantam Books, Inc.), 1975, p. 30.
[2]Ibid.

It was Alexander the Great who said:

I am dying
with the help
of too many physicians.

And it was Voltaire who remarked:

Doctors pour drugs
  of which they know little,
to cure diseases
  of which they know less,
into human beings
  of whom they know nothing.

Which brings me to the point of this chapter . . . that perhaps the medical profession should examine itself and the ethics and aspirations of its founder, Hippocrates.

Prevention Instead of Treatment

Perhaps, also, it should first devote more of its attention to the <u>prevention</u> of illness rather than to the <u>treatment</u>.

And perhaps the doctor should be paid on a monthly basis for his ability to keep his clients <u>well</u> and a deduction from his monthly income be made if they get sick!

Is this too radical a thought to project to the AMA?

Well, I can always go back to growing parsley (instead of writing books)!

7

DOES THE BIBLE APPROVE OF FASTING?

There are at least 15 specific instances where people fasted in the Bible.

And they went on a fast for different reasons. These instances and the reasons are listed briefly in a chart found in this chapter.

Sometimes instead of the word "fast," the descriptive phrase

to afflict the soul

is used. This often refers to physical fasting along with the accompanying spiritual humiliation. See Leviticus 16:29-31 as an example.

The only fast required by Moses was the yearly fast on the Day of Atonement.

After the Babylonian Captivity of the Israelites four annual fasts were held. This was in memory of the national calamities through which their nation had passed.

Israelites practiced both partial and total fasts.

The fast on the Day of Atonement was from evening to evening. See Leviticus 23:32. No food or drink was taken. Other fasts lasted from morning till evening.

Daniel Fasted 3 Weeks

Daniel fasted three full weeks after having a vision during the reign of Cyrus, King of Persia. The vision revealed a future time of great tribulation, wars and sorrow. See Daniel 10:1-3.

It cannot be said that fasts were always religious in nature. They were, however, perhaps as commonplace in Bible days as popping an aspirin is today. The difference, of course, is that fasting often produced more beneficial results than today's aspirins.

8 Occasions For Fasting

There are at least 8 notable biblical occasions on which fasting was practiced.

Private Afflictions

1 Samuel 1:7

Elkanah had two wives, Hannah and Peninnah. Peninnah had children. But Hannah was unable to bear any children. Peninnah taunted Hannah because of her barrenness.

Hannah had all she could take. She could not bear any more scoffing and ridicule.

She was so angry that she wept . . . and would not eat!

She went to the Tabernacle, where Eli, the priest was sitting in his place at the entrance.

And the Bible says:

> . . . she made a vow and said, "O Lord of hosts, if Thou wilt indeed look on the affliction of Thy maidservant and remember me, and not forget Thy

maidservant, but wilt thou give Thy
maidservant a son, then I will give him
to the Lord all the days of his life, and a
razor shall never come on his head."
(1 Samuel 1:11)

And what happend?

Then Eli answered and said, "Go in
peace; and may the God of Israel grant
your petition that you have asked of
Him."
And Elkanah knew Hannah, his wife,
and the Lord remembered her.
And it came about in due time, after
Hannah had conceived, that she gave
birth to a son; and she named him
Samuel, saying, "Because I have
asked him of the Lord."
(1 Samuel 1:17,19,20)

If you look closely at this illustration, Hannah did three very wise things.

First, she wept. And her weeping unleashed her pent-up emotions. All of us should at times weep. It is good for the soul as well as for the body.

Second, she fasted. This heightened her mental alertness and helped her cease her anger and desire for spiteful action into a more positive approach to her problem.

Third, but really the most important, she prayed. And God, in His infinite wisdom, answered her prayer.

It is not by accident that prayer and fasting are often mentioned together in the Bible.

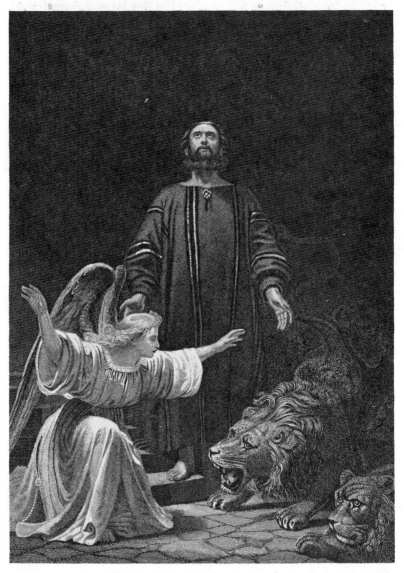

Darius, ruler of Babylon (539-525 B.C.), placed Daniel in the lions'
den. Darius, distressed at his dilemma, fasted. And God delivered
Daniel from all harm.

Public Disasters
(1 Samuel 31:11-13)
Saul and his three sons, including Jonathan, were killed in the battle against the Philistines. When Israelites from the tribe of Manasseh heard what the Philistines had done, they took the bodies of Saul and his sons and brought them to Jabesh where they were cremated. Then they fasted for seven days because of this tragedy.

Grief
(2 Samuel 12:16)
You will recall David murdered Uriah and stole his wife, Bathsheba. She had a baby by David. The baby became desperately ill. David fasted. On the seventh day of his fast, the baby died.

Upon being told the baby died, he washed himself, changed his clothes, and went into the Tabernacle and worshiped the Lord. His aides were amazed and asked him:

> . . . While the child was alive,
> you fasted and wept;
> but when the child died,
> you arose and ate food.

They could not understand this action. David replied:

> While the child was still alive,
> I fasted and wept;
> for I said, Who knows,
> the Lord may be gracious to me,
> that the child may live.

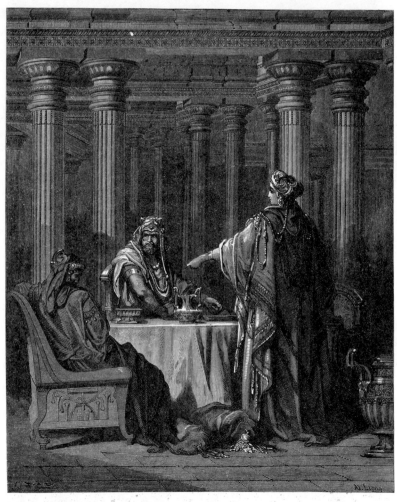

Queen Esther, concerned that her people would soon die because of the wicked intrigue of Haman, prime minister of Persia . . . asked all the Jews in Susa to fast for three days.

Esther then brought Haman and King Ahasuerus together at a banquet. At this banquet she points the finger of accusation at Haman. And God honored the prayer and fasting of His people. Haman was hanged on gallows he had built for Mordecai.

> But now he has died;
> why should I fast?
> Can I bring him back again?

God does not always grant a prayer while fasting. He did honor Hannah's request for a child, but not David's request to save the life of his child.

Anxiety

(Daniel 6:18-20)

When Darius, because of the laws of the Medes and the Persians, had to place his friend Daniel in the lions' den . . . he was very distressed. That night he spent in fasting.

Just prior to fasting, Darius told Daniel:

> Your God whom you constantly serve
> will Himself deliver you.
> (Daniel 6:16)

And Darius fasted. And God did deliver Daniel!

Approaching Danger

(Esther 4:16)

King Ahasuerus, through the guile of his prime minister Haman, signed a decree that all the Jews, young and old, women and children, must all be killed on the 28th day of February of the following year.

He also decreed that their property was to be given to those who killed them.

When Queen Esther heard about this she told Mordecai, her cousin:

Go, assemble all the Jews
who are found in Susa,
and fast for me;
do not eat or drink for three days,
night or day.

I and my maidens also
will fast in the same way.
And thus I will go in to the king,
which is not according to the law;
and
if I perish, I perish. (Esther 4:16-17)

And they did fast. And God did hear their cry and saved them!

National Repentance
(1 Samuel 7:5-6)

The people of Israel had wandered far from the Lord. All Israel was in sorrow because it appeared that the Lord had abandoned them for a period of some 20 years.

Samuel reminded the Israelites that if they were really serious about returning to the Lord they should get rid of their foreign gods and idols. The Philistines had been successful in their forays against God's people but Samuel reminded them that if they repented, God would rescue them from this oppression.

And they gathered to Mizpah,
and drew water
and poured it out before the Lord,
and fasted on that day,
and said there,
"We have sinned against the Lord."
(1 Samuel 7:6)

And God heard their prayer. And God did deliver them from the Philistines!

Sad News
Nehemiah 1:4

In December of the 20th year of the reign of King Artaxerxes of Persia, while Nehemiah was at the palace of Shushan, he received some bad news.

A fellow Jew, Hanani, having just arrived from Judah, told him that things were not going well in Jerusalem. The walls of Jerusalem were still torn down and the gates were burned.

Nehemiah, upon hearing this:

> . . . wept and mourned for days;
> and I was fasting and praying
> before the God of heaven.
> . . . I and my father's house
>   have sinned.
> We have acted corruptly against Thee
> and have not kept the commandments,
> nor the statutes, nor the ordinances
> which Thou didst command
>   Thy servant Moses.
> O Lord, I beseech Thee,
> may Thine ear be attentive
> to the prayer of Thy servant and
> the prayer of Thy servants
> who delight to revere Thy name
> and make Thy servant successful today,
> and grant him compassion before
>   this man.
> (Nehemiah 1:4,6,7,11)

And God heard Nehemiah's prayer. When Nehemiah appeared before King Artaxerxes and asked permission to take a

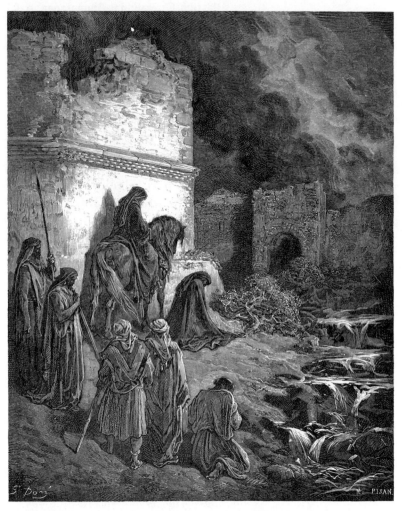

In 445 B.C. Nehemiah, a Jewish patriot and Persian statesman, concerned about the disintegration of Jerusalem . . . prayed and fasted. Then he approached King Artaxerxes and asked permission to take a leave of absence and rebuild the walls of Jerusalem. The King agreed!

leave of absence to rebuild Jerusalem, the King agreed.

Sacred Ordination
(Acts 13:3)

Among the prophets and teachers at the Church at Antioch were Paul and Barnabas.

> And while they were ministering
>   to the Lord
> and fasting,
> the Holy Spirit said,
> "Set apart for Me Barnabas and Saul
> for the work
> to which I have called them."
> Then, when they had fasted
> and prayed
> and laid their hands on them,
> they sent them away.
>   (Acts:13:2-3)

Here we see an example of fasting used as a part of God's ordination on a ministry. Should such an example be also followed today?

Does the Bible Approve?

Perhaps you may ask the question: "Does the Bible approve of fasting?"

And it might be best to answer in the negative. The Bible certainly does not disapprove of fasting. And the Bible cites many examples of fasting both for physical and spiritual reasons.

Fasts in the Bible have been as short as one day (Judges 20:26), or one night (Daniel 6;18) to as long as 40 days. Moses (Exodus 34:28), Elijah (1 Kings 19:8) and Jesus (Matthew 4:2) fasted 40 days. A word of caution, however, fasting of more than three days should NOT be done without the care and supervision of your physician.

When the men of Bethel questioned the validity of their fasts Zechariah reminded them that obedience, justice and kindness were equally as important as fasting. If they fasted but did not repent of their ways and did not obey God's commands their fasting would be ineffectual. See Zechariah 7.

The fasts, God reminded them, were to be seasons of inward joy (Zechariah 8:19).

Anna served God with fasting (Luke 2:37).

Certain demons could only be cast out by prayer and fasting (Matthew 17:21—Some Bibles omit this last word because it was absent from the oldest manuscripts).

Paul fasted following his vision on the road to Damascus (Acts 9:9).

Those on the storm-tossed ship with Paul fasted for 14 days (Acts 27:33).

And if you will look at the chart in this chapter you will see other instances of fasting by prophets and apostles.

Does God approve of fasting?

All indications in Scripture lead me to believe that fasting was a valid form of spiritual and physical cleansing.

And I personally believe it should be practiced today.

This was a most difficult chapter to write. But I wrote it while on a 24-hour fast.

And even though the subject matter is difficult, I was able to complete it with ease and clarity of mind while fasting!

5 Guidelines when Fasting

Scriptures give us five guidelines when fasting.

1. Remember God (Zechariah 7)

2. Chasten the soul

> When I wept in my soul
> with fasting,
> It became my reproach. (Psalm 69:10)

3. Humble the soul

> Malicious witnesses rise up;
> They repay me evil for good . . .
> I humbled myself
> with fasting . . .   (Psalm 35:11-13)

4. Avoid display

At the time of Christ's Sermon on the Mount, He offered this advice:

> . . . whenever you fast,
> do not put on a gloomy face
> as the hypocrites do,
> for they neglect their appearance
> in order to be seen fasting by men.
>
> Truly I say to you,
> they have their reward in full.
>
> But you, when you fast,
> anoint your head,
> and wash your face
> so that you may not be seen
>   fasting by men,
> but by your Father who is
>   in secret;
> and your Father
> who sees in secret
> will reward thee openly.
>   (Matthew 6:16-18)

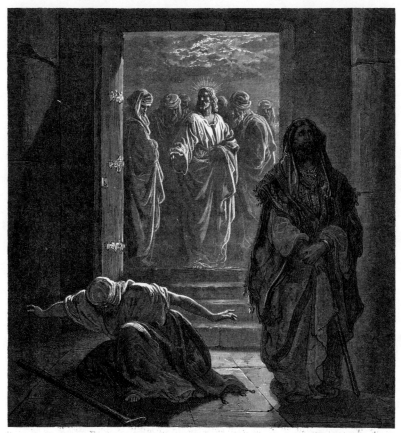

Fasting and prayer should be done in meekness and humbleness not in boastful public display. Remember the Pharisee who went into the temple to pray with the tax collector [publican] ? In Luke 18:12, the Pharisee boasts: *"I fast twice in the week; I give tithes of all that I possess."*

Further he stated, *"I thank thee that I am not as other men are . . . even as this tax collector"* (Luke 18:11).

"And the tax collector, standing afar off, would not lift up so much as his eyes unto heaven, but smote upon his breast, saying, God be merciful to me a sinner" (Luke 18:13).

Christ reminds us: *". . .every one who exalts himself will be humbled, but he who humbles himself will be exalted"* (Luke 18:14).

". . . do not put on a gloomy face as the hypocrites do. . . ." With all the gloomy faces one sometimes sees in Bible-believing churches one wonders if the church is plagued with hypocrites???

5. Consider the true meaning of fasting

There is a right reason and a wrong reason for fasting and Isaiah reminded the people of Israel that they were fasting for the wrong reason when they asked:

> Why have we fasted
> and thou dost not see?
> Why have we humbled ourselves
> and thou dost not notice?
> (Isaiah 58:3)

The prophet Isaiah, in righteous indignation, replied:

> Behold, you fast for contention
> and strife
> and to strike with a wicked fist.
> (Isaiah 58:4)

He reminds them that they should fast:

> To loosen the bonds of wickedness,
> To undo the bands of the yoke,
> And let the oppressed go free . . .
> To divide your bread with the hungry,
> And bring the homeless poor
> into the house;
> When you see the naked, to cover him;
> And not to hide yourself from your
> own flesh.
> (Isaiah 58:6-7)

Then, if they follow this he promises:

Then your light
will break out like dawn,
And your recovery
will speedily spring forth;
And your righteousness
will go before you;
The glory of the Lord
will be your rear guard.
Then you will call,
and the Lord will answer!

(Isaiah 58:8-9)

What a message for each of us today! If those in the church would stop their contention, if we would show real, honest concern for the hungry and the poor in our congregation and show real love for members of our own family . . . what blessings God would outpour on us.

And it all can begin with sincere, humble fasting! Are you ready for such a revival in your own heart and life?

Person	Scripture Reference	Length of Fast	Reason for Fasting	Outcome of Fasting
Moses	Exodus 34:27,28	40 days and 40 nights	He fasted during the holy period of being in God's presence on Mt. Sinai.	The Lord gave the Ten Commandments to Moses and the children of Israel.
The sons of Israel and all the people	Judges 20,26	All the sons of Israel and all the people went up to Bethel ("House-of-God") to fast from after their second day of defeat until evening.	They wanted to know if they should go out to battle against the sons of Benjamin for a third time.	The Lord delivered the sons of Benjamin into the hands of the sons of Israel in the third battle.
The sons of Israel	1 Samuel 7:5,6	One day	The sons of Israel confessed their sin of idolatry to the Lord.	While the sons of Israel fasted, the Philistines prepared for battle against Israel. Samuel prayed to the Lord, who answered him by sending great thunder which routed the Philistines. The men of Israel then pursued the Philistines and regained their land. The Lord continued to protect Israel from the Philistines all the days of Samuel.
David	2 Samuel 12:16	Seven days (?)	David fasted and prayed for the Lord to let his child live.	The child died

Person	Scripture Reference	Length of Fast	Reason for Fasting	Outcome of Fasting
Elijah	1 Kings 19:8	40 days and 40 nights	The angel of the Lord provided Elijah with two meals that gave him enough strength to travel without additional food for 40 days and 40 nights from Jezreel to Horeb.	Elijah reached Horeb, the mountain of God, and received encouragement and instructions from the Lord.
The King, nobles and people of Nineveh	Jonah 3:5-8	Unspecified	The people fasted in repentance of their sin and asked God for help to turn from their wicked ways.	The people of Nineveh turned from their wicked ways and God did not punish them.
Nehemiah	Nehemiah 1:4	Unspecified	Nehemiah mourned for the exiles and the condition of Jerusalem, confessed his sin and the sin of the sons of Israel, and fasted in God's presence in preparation for his requesting King Artaxerxes to permit him to rebuild Jerusalem.	King Artaxerxes granted Nehemiah permission to go to Jerusalem to rebuild the city.
King Darius	Daniel 6:18	One night — evening (sunset) to morning (sunrise)	Darius fasted while Daniel was in the lions' den, believing Daniel's God could deliver him from the lions.	God kept Daniel safe, and Darius ordered Daniel's accusers and their wives and children to be cast into the lions' den. Darius made a decree that all people in his kingdom were to fear and tremble before the God of Daniel.

Person	Scripture Reference	Length of Fast	Reason for Fasting	Outcome of Fasting
Daniel	Daniel 9:3	Unspecified	Daniel fasted to confess the sin of all Israel. He asked God to turn His anger away from Jerusalem, and to forgive his people.	Gabriel gave Daniel the great prophecy of the Seventy Weeks.
Anna	Luke 2:36-38	The length of her fasts are not given but she fasted and prayed often in the Temple.	Anna served God by her frequent fasting and devotion to prayer.	Anna's devotion to God led her to speak of the birth of the Christ-child to "all those who looked for redemption in Jerusalem."
Jesus	Matthew 4:1,2	40 days and 40 nights	Jesus was "led up by the Spirit into the wilderness to be tested by the devil."	Satan was unsuccessful. Jesus' victory illustrates the Scripture in Hebrews 4:14,15, ". . . Jesus, the Son of God . . . was in all points tempted like as we are, yet without sin."
Apostles	2 Corinthians 6:4,5	Unspecified	Various fastings during Paul and his associates' ministry, as well as times when necessity forced them to go without eating.	A fruitful ministry before God, and a good testimony before all.
Early Christians	Acts 13:2,3	Unspecified	They may have been seeking the Lord's will on the question of missions. The Holy Spirit spoke to them as they ministered to the Lord and fasted. After setting apart Barnabas and Saul, the early Christians again fasted and then prayed and laid their hands on them.	The Holy Spirit sent forth Barnabas and Saul on the first missionary journey.

8

GIVE ME 7 GOOD REASONS FOR FASTING

There is a Hasidic saying that

*A man must not rely on pure reason;
he must mix faith with it.*

When a judge asked an individual a reason for a certain action, the reply was:

I am a woman, I haven't any.

But, seriously, there are very good reasons for fasting! And they will be covered in this chapter.

What is Fasting?

First, understand this: fasting is NOT starving! Fasting does not exhaust the body's reserves. If fasting is continued past a tolerable limit and the body's reserves are used up, then starving begins.

There is quite a difference between fasting and starving. Thousands of people have fasted, under medical supervision, 25-30 days. And many more thousands fast 24 hours each week.

In Europe, fasting has long been accepted by reputable doctors. The Buchinger Sanatorium in Bad Pyrmont, Germany, has supervised more than 70,000 fasts.

**Fasting
Clinics**

Fasting clinics are scattered through Sweden, France, Switzerland and Norway. Over 30,000 fasts have been conducted by Herbert Shelton in San Antonio, Texas. And more than 15,000 fasters have visited the Pawling Health Manor near Hyde Park, New York.

When you fast, in the strict sense of the word, you consume only water. NO FOOD. In fact, water is a faster's best friend. In a sense, fasting is the absence of food from one's diet and the absence of all liquids except water.

**How Does
the Fasting
Process
Work?**

In the previous chapters we have shown you how you assimilate some 4 pounds of chemical preservatives and additives a year.

And by injudicious eating you probably consume gallons of soft drinks, many pounds of sugar through cakes, pies and candy and have built up your cholesterol level and increased your blood pressure.

And your digestive system, including your liver and kidneys, become the whipping boys, having to work overtime to clean the wastes you have dumped into your body.

**Your
Miracle Kidneys**

Your kidneys are a miracle working machine. They are equipped with filtering, absorbing and secreting units called nephrons. Your body has about 2½ million nephrons and, if all their tubules were straightened out, they would stretch for approximately 50 miles!

Outside of the brain, the kidneys are perhaps the most complex organ of the body.

Now, when you go on a fast, you allow the digestive systems in your body to rest.

Thus the cleansing capacity of the lungs, the liver, the kidneys and the skin are intensified. The accumulated toxins in your body from food additives and indiscreet eating, when in a fast, are released into the bloodstream and then expelled.

The Value of Water

Water is the great flushing agent in fasting, getting rid of the toxins and waste materials that build up when fatty tissue is "burned."

When on a fast, a sure sign that these poisons are being eliminated can be seen in the concentration of toxins in the urine. These toxins may be 10 times higher than normal.

Another sign of toxic elimination is that you will notice a coating on your tongue.

Fasting is not a cure for disease. Fasting gives your digestive organs a rest so that its energies can be devoted to cleansing your body of impurities. This cleansing also according to the testimony of thousands who do fast, eliminates some of the causes of illness.

Fasting Eliminates Toxins

When you make your stomach a garbage can ... your heart suffers, your arteries suffer, you poison your blood stream.

This is sometimes called autointoxication. This is a condition caused by poisonous substances produced within the body. Fasting quickly stops this intake of decomposition-toxins and then gives the organism a chance to catch up with its work of excretion. It helps remove toxins in the tissues. And it causes the body to consume its excess of fat.

As these wastes are eliminated during your fast, you will find you have increased energy, a keener alertness, and you should have a brighter disposition towards life. With poisons eliminated, your entire outlook should change. Depression, anxiety, worry somehow fade into the horizon.

Fasting ...
A Valid
Remedy

Dr. Allan Cott, a New York City psychiatrist, says:

The empirical data from people who say they were cured by fasting is not acceptable in medical journals ...

But under the supervision of hygienists, many sick people have fasted and recovered from really serious ailments — after their doctors had all but given up on them.

The medical profession is so tuned in to "curing" by introducing drugs into the system it cannot accept the idea that by eliminating everything the body can go about healing itself.

Yet the system apparently works for animals, who go off and rest without eating when wounded or ill. Fasting is certainly not a panacea for all ills, but it may be effective in treating many more varieties of sickness than orthodox medicine is ever likely to concede.[1]

---

[1]Allan Cott, M.D., Fasting: The Ultimate Diet, (New York: Bantam Books, Inc.), 1975, pp. 15,16.

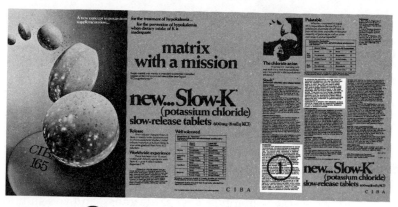

In the September 10, 1975 issue of *Medical Tribune* appeared a 4-page full color ad insert on Slow-K tablets, a slow-release potassium chloride tablet given to supply potassium when diuretics are administered to the patient. [Diuretics often have a tendency to deplete the body of its potassium.]

The Medical letter, a non-profit publication on Drugs and Therapeutics, in their August 29, 1975 issue states: ***"Slow-release potassium tablets such as Slow-K . . . are dangerous and should not be used."*** They wisely recommend the patient eat two medium-sized bananas plus one eight-ounce glass of orange juice to replace potassium loss.

I Would Hear of a Faster

I had known about fasting for some time. I am now 49 years of age. And only now have I begun fasting. Actually, as I am writing this chapter, I am on a 24-hour fast. I began yesterday after breakfast. It is now 10 AM the following morning. And I will break my fast at noon with a salad of raw carrots and grated cabbage.

From time to time, I would hear of someone who was fasting, such as the late Mahatma Ghandi, prisoners who went on protest fasts, and Paul Bragg, who at 85, wrote, The Miracle of Fasting.

That Week in the Philippines

About 10 years ago, I traveled for 2 years with a well-known evangelist in Crusades overseas in the Holy land and in the Philippines. I noticed that he had what appeared to be an inexhaustible supply of energy. In the heat of the Philippine day, he would preach for more than an hour with a shirt and tie and coat on. By the end of the message he was literally dripping in perspiration.

And I was exhausted just watching him. But the next day he would be bright and bouncy. While I was dragging myself around and fatigued.

I heard that he prayed and fasted regularly. When he ate, I believe he only ate one meal a day on these crusades and that was usually fresh fruit and salads. When he ate, I would eat hamburgers. And I would be tired by nightfall while he would still be fresh and alert.

**A Chance
Discussion
and
4 Pounds Lost**

That was some 10 years ago. Since then the subject of fasting was only a fleeting interest to me at rare intervals.

Then, in August, 1975, my wife happened to pick up a popular magazine in which was included an article on fasting. At the dinner table quite a discussion on fasting ensued.

On the spur of the moment, I suggested: "Let's try a 24-hour fast this week."

And that's when my wife and I started to fast. That's how I developed an interest in the subject . . . began researching it and found it to be both fascinating and beneficial.

In the first 24-hour fast, my wife lost 5 pounds; I lost 4 pounds. Both of us felt more alive, more alert. And both of us slept soundly!

**Give Me 7
Good Reasons
for Fasting**

It's not hard to give you 7 good reasons for fasting, because there are many more than 7 reasons why fasting can be beneficial to you.

But here are some:

1. To lower your blood pressure
2. To lower your cholesterol level
3. To clean out your body
4. To give your digestive system a rest
5. To give your body time to heal itself
6. To relieve nervousness and tension
7. To sleep better
8. To regulate your bowels providing better elimination
9. To make you more alert

10. To sharpen your mental processes
11. To slow your aging process
12. To save money
13. To feel and look better physically
14. To lose weight, quick and easy
15. To improve your marital life
16. To help you eliminate smoking and drinking
17. To learn the will of God

Now that last reason, if for no other reason, is a valid reason for fasting.

Fasting Brings A New Consecration

Andrew Murray, a spiritual giant, and a missionary to Africa in the last century, believed in fasting. He wrote:

> Learn from these men [Those in the Church at Antioch; Acts 13] that the work which the Holy Ghost commands must call us to new fasting and prayer, to new separation from the spirit and the pleasures of the world, to new consecration to God and to His fellowship.
>
> Those men gave themselves up to fasting and prayer, and if in all our ordinary Christian work there were more prayer there would be more blessing in our own inner life.[1]

There are many other reasons for fasting.

The Royal Road to Healing

Dr. Otto H.F. Buchinger, who has supervised more than 70,000 fasts, states:

> Fasting is . . . a royal road to healing for anyone who agrees to take it for the recovery and regeneration of the body,

---

[1]Andrew Murray, Full and Joyous Surrender (Westchester, Illinois: Good News Publishers), 1959, p.20.

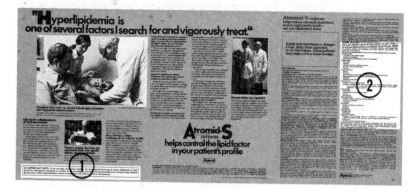

AN IMPORTANT NOTE: It has not been established whether the drug-induced lowering of serum cholesterol or lipid levels has a detrimental, beneficial, or no effect on the morbidity or mortality due to atherosclerosis or coronary heart disease. Several years will be required before current investigations will yield an answer to this question.

ADVERSE REACTIONS: Of the pertinent reactions, the most common is nausea. Less frequently encountered gastrointestinal reactions are vomiting, loose stools, dyspepsia, flatulence, and abdominal distress. Reactions reported less often than gastrointestinal ones are headache, dizziness, and fatigue; muscle cramping, aching, and weakness; skin rash, urticaria, and pruritus; dry brittle hair, and alopecia.

The following reported adverse reactions are listed alphabetically by systems:

Cardiovascular
  Increased or decreased angina
  Cardiac arrhythmias
  Both swelling and phlebitis at site of xanthomas
Dermatologic
  Skin rash
  Alopecia
  Allergic reaction including urticaria
  Dry skin and dry brittle hair
  Pruritus
Gastrointestinal
  Nausea
  Diarrhea
  Gastrointestinal upset (bloating, flatulence, abdominal distress)
  Hepatomegaly (not associated with hepatotoxicity)
  Vomiting
  Stomatitis and gastritis
Genitourinary
  Impotence and decreased libido
  Findings consistent with renal dysfunction as evidenced by dysuria, hematuria, proteinuria, decreased urine output. One patient's renal biopsy suggested "allergic reaction."
Hematologic
  Leukopenia
  Potentiation of anticoagulant effect
  Anemia
  Eosinophilia
Musculoskeletal
  Myalgia (muscle cramping, aching, weakness)
  "Flu like" symptoms
  Arthralgia
Neurologic
  Fatigue, weakness, drowsiness
  Dizziness
  Headache
Miscellaneous
  Weight gain
  Polyphagia
Laboratory Findings
  Abnormal liver function tests as evidenced by increased transaminase (SGOT and SGPT), BSP retention, and increased thymol turbidity
  Proteinuria
  Increased creatine phosphokinase

Reported adverse reactions whose direct relationship with the drug has not been established: peptic ulcer, gastrointestinal hemorrhage, rheumatoid arthritis, tremors, increased perspiration, systemic lupus erythematosus, blurred vision, gynecomastia, thrombocytopenic purpura.

mind and spirit.[1]

Dr. Buchinger feels the following illnesses, among others, merit fasting:

1. Overweight
2. Rheumatism in the joints and muscles
3. Diseases of the heart, circulation and blood vessels, such as: high or low blood pressure; hot flashes
4. Stress and nervous exhaustion
5. Skin diseases
6. Diseases of the digestive organs
7. Diseases of the respiratory organs
8. Kidney and bladder disease
9. Female complaints
10. Allergies, such as hay fever
11. Eye diseases such as chronic iritis, retinitis

**Consult
Your Doctor**

May I once again remind you, it is the purpose of this book solely to introduce you to the concept of fasting. Nothing in this book is intended to constitute medical treatment or advice of any nature.

Before any fast, you should consult your medical doctor. This is particularly true of fasts that last longer than 24 hours.

One of the unusual benefits of fasting is that fasting SAVES TIME!

---

[1]Otto H.F. Buchinger, M.D., Everything You Want to Know About Fasting (New York: Pyramid Books), 1972, Forward.

**Fasting
Saves
Time**

Have you ever counted up the minutes you spend each day in eating?

I generally go out for breakfast in order to read the newspaper and take a break . . . since I work at home all day . . . in writing and research.	Time for Breakfast 1 Hour
Mary and I usually have lunch at home.	Time for Lunch 40 Minutes
Our family has dinner	Time for Dinner 40 Minutes
Before we go to bed we generally have a snack	Time for Snack 30 Minutes

Now, if you add that all up . . . you will find just in eating and sitting around the table we have used up 170 minutes of our time a day . . . or almost 3 hours!

Three hours a day to eat. And more for my wife, because she has to clean off the table and wash the dishes and put them away after each meal!

When we fast, we have a glass of distilled water for our meal. This takes about 1 minute.

In a day of fasting we have used 3-5 minutes while in a day of eating, we have expended 3 hours!

What a difference.

**3 Hours
Saved!**

All of a sudden we found we had 3 hours on our hands each fast day. These "found" hours were put to work productively. Mary and I took walks, got to know each other better. We had sweet fellowship walking hand in hand around our community. We went shopping together. And I was able to devote more time to writing with a sharper, more clear mind.

We became more aware of food, too. It would seem everytime we turned on the TV, there was a food commercial. Our senses sharpened. While on a fast, the aroma from Mary's cooking for our children . . . seemed to always waft past my nose.

Think of it . . . save 3 hours each day by fasting. You often said, "Oh, if there were just more hours in the day!"

I've just found you THREE! Now, go and make them productive!

Well, my 24-hour fast is over. Guess I'll go into the kitchen and whip up a scrumptious salad.

And no, I won't forget the parsley!

NUGGETS OF TRUTH

One of the important reasons for fasting is that it gives your body a rest. This is rest of the glandular, digestive, circulatory, respiratory and nervous systems. When you abstain from food, the glands of the mouth and stomach, the liver and pancreas . . . rest. This rest provides an opportunity for your body to do for itself what it cannot do under conditions of full activity.

* * *

Some fasting clinics have discovered that, contrary to popular belief, invalids who fast have experienced a gain of strength, instead of losing it!

Fasting and Arthritis

Dr. Herbert M. Shelton has conducted over 30,000 fasts. In his book, *Fasting Can Save Your Life*, He makes the following comments:

Rheumatic arthritis, as distinguished from traumatic and tubercular arthritis, represents an impaired state of nutrition in addition to the common toxemia . . . To be truly effective the care of the arthritic case should be directed at the removal of the cause of the disease. To give drugs . . . is to remove no cause.

Fasting relieves the pains of arthritis, for example, more effectively than drugs and does it without risk or harm . . .

It is customary to advise the arthritic to exercise the affected joints to prevent these from becoming fixed. It is asserted that this stays the development of ankylosis or bony union. However much truth there may be in this claim, the forced activity tends to aggravate the inflammation and intensify the pain. I find it better to let the affected join rest until fasting has enabled the body to remove the deposits and infiltrations from the joint and to clear up the inflammation. In this way the stiff joint spontaneously limbers up and may be used without pain.[1]

Dr. Shelton believes that many forms of standard methods of treatment with drugs have left the patient progressively worse.

---

[1]

Herbert M. Shelton, *Fasting Can Save Your Life* (Chicago: Natural Hygiene Press),, 1973, pp. 122-124.

Fasting and the Peptic Ulcer

Peptic ulcers generally reveal that in the very early life of the patient he has developed a gastro-intestinal irritation and inflammation. This has been perhaps caused by his unbalanced mode of living and eating.

From this stage of irritation then comes inflammation and gradual thickening of the mucous and sub-mucous tissues, and then ulceration.

The increased hardening chokes arterial circulation. This cuts off oxygen and the food supply. The tissues break down giving rise to an open sore or ulcer. An ulcer is an ending in a chain of symptoms.

Some believe that the patient should eat every three or four hours. The danger in this is that the patient overeats causing excess secretion to be continued which aggravates the situation and does not correct it.

Milk diets, bland diets and small meals alleviate the symptoms but do not remove the cause!

Too many physicians are quick to recommend surgery. The first step necessary to insure healing of a peptic ulcer is complete rest for the ulcerated organ. Nothing gives the digestive organs a more complete rest than the fast. Fasting causes a cessation of secretion of gastric juice. Thus this source of irritation is removed by the fast.

The fast removes three sources of local irritation: the *mechanical irritation* brought on by particles of food that come in contact with the raw surface, the mechanical irritation which results from *contraction and expansion* of the walls of the stomach and *wrinkling of its surfaces* in receiving and handling foods, and chemical irritation caused by the acid gastric juice. These observations are made by Dr. Herbert M. Shelton.

Dr. Shelton believes that the fast must be continued, under medical supervision, until all reactions indicate that systemic renovation have been completed. Fasting, however, will not result in a removal of scar tissue.

* * *

Fasting and Hay Fever

Hay fever can be described as a chronic inflammation of the nasal passages growing out of a pronounced toxemic condition that perhaps has lasted for years.

Toxemia is distribution throughout the body of poisonous products of bacteria growing in a focal or local site, thus producing generalized symptoms. So long as this toxemic state is maintained by such things as overeating, there is no possibility of recovering from hay fever.

If you abstain from food for a time you may notice that the nasal discharge and other symptoms of hay fever clear up. I have!

Fasting and the Heart

Some engaged in conducting fasting clinics report that instead of fasting weakening the heart, it results in *strengthening* this wonderful organ!

Dr. Herbert M. Shelton reports:

> In the hundreds of cases of heart disease that I have watched through fasts of various lengths, all but a few have developed stronger and better hearts. Many of them, even so-called incurable ones, have become entirely normal.

> Rapid hearts have slowed down, abnormally slow hearts have speeded up, weak hearts have greatly improved in vigor, hearts that were irregular have become regular in time and frequency, hearts that were missing pulsations have resumed regular pulsation. . . .

> Since fasting relieves the heart of a great burden, improvement should not be surprising.[1]

Fasting gives the heart a rest from its digestive functions allowing it greater opportunity to repair itself and renew its functional vigor. As an example, a heart that is pulsating 80 times a minute may fall to 60 or even fewer beats per minute. A saving of 20 fewer beats per minute is 1200 per hour. And in just 24 hours your heart, by fasting saves 28,800 pulsations. In other words, your heart has to beat 28,800 times **LESS** thus reducing the work load on your heart!

---

[1]

Herbert M. Shelton, *Fasting Can Save Your Life* (Chicago: Natural Hygiene Press), 1973, p. 143.

Fasting and Colitis

Colitis is inflammation of the colon.

The human colon (large bowel) is divided into three sections:

ascending
transverse
descending

The most annoying symptom of colitis is constipation. This is sometimes alternated with diarrhea.

Many people who suffer from chronic colitis are rarely cheerful or happy. They sometimes have what is called a "colon complex," which is a negative or depressive psychosis. Depressive psychosis is defined as being characterized by extreme depression, melancholia, and feelings of unworthiness.

Often in colitis, the facial expression is one of dejection and misery. The individual may become very nervous, irritable and even border on hysteria.

Colitis sufferers complain of indigestion, rumbling of gas in the intestines. Many times they suffer from a constant dull headache.

The continual irritation of the bowels by drugging only leads to the suffering of the patient. Yet how many feel that drugs and patent medicine are the cure-all to their problem!

Fasting speeds up that part of metabolism that eliminates waste. Fasting also rejuvenates fatigued nerve and cell structure. Physicians who recommend a liberal diet, barbiturates to aid sleep at night, and tincture of belladonna or phenobarbital to quiet the bowels . . . should seriously reexamine their procedures.

Fasting could be the answer to giving more lasting and more beneficial results.

Fasting and the Prostate Gland

The prostate is a gland which surrounds the neck of the bladder and the urethra in the male. It is partly glandular, with ducts opening into the prostatic portion of the urethra, and partly muscular.

Enlargement of the prostate is common in men after middle age. This results in urethral obstruction, impeding urination and sometimes leading to retention of urine in the bladder. Benign and malignant tumors are common, particularly in men past 60.

Physicians often recommend surgery for removal (or partial removal) of the prostate gland. Such radical measures are, in the opinion of the author, highly unsatisfactory. The patient is sometimes worse off after the operation than before.

Overeating, tea, coffee, tobacco, alcohol and other stimulants contribute to the enlargement of the prostate.

In his fasting clinic, Dr. Shelton has seen prostate glands that were as large as baseballs (and nearly as hard) reduced to a normal size in a week after fasting. The hardness was entirely dissolved, so that urination was normal after proper care was given.

Fasting does not cure problems of the prostate. Fasting does allow the natural healing powers of the body to function. But if you return to overeating and taking of stimulants the prostate will quickly be aggravated to its former condition.

Fasting and Gallstones

Choleitiasis is the formation or presence of calculi or bile-stones in the gallbladder or common duct.

Generally the core of all gallstones contains a mixture of cholesterol, bilirubin [the orange colored pigment in bile] and protein. The stone may remain dormant and give little distress unless inflammation and distention of the gallbladder take place or unless it enters and is unable to pass through the biliary ducts. Then colic ensues.

Hospital treatment generally consists of morphine for initial colic attacks. The standard treatment for gallstone problems is surgical removal of the gallbladder.

Yet patients who have their gallbladder removed are usually warned by their physician that such surgery will not remove the symptoms of bloating, belching and upper abdominal discomfort.

In fact, the 12th edition of the Merck Manual, published by Merck Sharp & Dohme Research Laboratories, states on page 785:

There is no known medical treatment for gallstones.

Stone formation may be caused by heavy eating of carbohydrate foods (sugars and starches) and lack of exercise.

Those who conduct fasting clinics report that a fast will enable the body to perform an excellent job of drainage and do it in a way to leave the gall bladder intact and unharmed. Certainly the patient is not restored to good health when his gallbladder is removed!

Dr. George S. Weger, who has had extensive experience with gallstones both as a physician and hygienist says:

Given proper assistance, the chemistry of the body can be so altered that stones soften, disintegrate and pass out with but slight discomfort.

Softening of gallstones occurs very rapidly when one is on a complete fast.

Those with gallstone problems should, after a fast, restrict their diet as much as possible with fresh fruits, fresh salads and cooked non-starchy vegetables.

Doctor Reports Fasting Benefits

In the September, 1975 issue of Prevention, pages 55-62, Dr. Bernie Rappaport of California reports that fasting is beneficial.

Dr. Rappaport is a medical doctor with a specialty in psychiatry and nutritional counseling. He believes that medicine, as usually practiced, is based almost entirely on the diagnosis of symptoms, once a disease has already been manifested.

He advocates preventive medicine.

He eats unprocessed, organically grown foods and only a minimum of meat, principally chicken and fish. He drinks herb teas rather than coffee and consumes most vegetables raw.

He believes that indigestion and recurrent infections will often respond positively to a cleansing fast, where the patient eats nothing but raw fruits and vegetables for a few days. Fruits and vegetables should not be mixed at the same meal, however, for they have a tendency of producing gas and indigestion.

Dr. Rappaport has fasted for as long as 10 days. He says: "Fasting is not the ordeal most people believe it to be . . . What you put into your body . . . has a lot to do with how you feel."

*   *   *

Fasting brings about a radical cleansing of the fluids and tissues of the body. However, it cannot prevent the subsequent fouling of these same fluids and tissues if you return to overeating patterns.

*   *   *

My associate, Bob Conner, tells me he is partial to parsley . . . that whenever he feels down and out . . . he eats parsley and he becomes "parsley revived!"

9

CAN I LOSE WEIGHT BY FASTING?

Columnist Hal Boyle once wrote:

When a 220-pound man laughs,
there is twice as much of him
having a good time
as when a 110-pound man laughs.
This is one of the advantages
of being fat.

There are few, very few advantages to being fat. And they are "outweighed" by a multiplicity of disadvantages!

One man suggested a good reducing exercise consisted of placing both hands against the dinner table edge and pushing back!

One of the common complications of obesity is damage to the cardiovascular system. Obesity, in laymen terms, is simply being overweight.

In the overweight person an abnormal amount of fat is on the body. The term "obesity" is usually applied to an individual when he is 20-30% over his average weight for his age, sex and height.

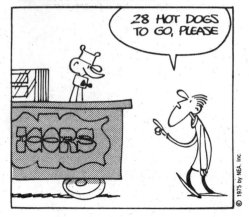
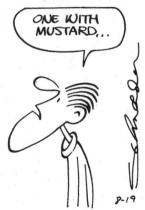
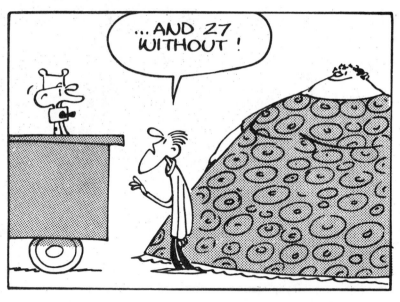

Obesity is the result of an imbalance

between the food eaten
and
energy expended

Two Causes

There are two general classifications of those being overweight:

1. Excessive food intake
2. That caused by some abnormality within the body

However, the main cause of obesity is in the first one listed — that is, eating more calories than are required to maintain normal body weight.

**Dangers
in Being
Overweight**

There are many disadvantages and dangers in being overweight.

1. Overweight people tend to have a shorter life-span.
2. Obesity has a tendency to make one more susceptible to diabetes, high blood pressure, heart failure, arteriosclerosis, gallbladder disease, varicose veins and hernia.
3. Obesity leads to shortness of breath and difficulty in sleeping.
4. Those overweight usually have more complaints on the intestinal tract such as indigestion, belching, flatulence and constipation.
5. Headache, fatigue and irritability are seen more frequently in obese people.

Many physicians believe that obesity in the early years of life tends to cause premature hardening of the arteries.

Those overweight also usually suffer more discomfort and pain from arthritis than thin people.

Life insurance statistics show that a person who weighs 10% more than he should may have a 20% shorter life expectancy than the person of normal weight. And the more the overweight, the higher the percentage of a shorter life expectancy.

There are many fad diets on the market. All cost money. There's the grapefruit diet, the vinegar-lecithin-kelp diet, the "quick-weight loss" diet, the "eat what you want and grow slim" diet, etc.

But the most practical way to lose weight and the least expensive is by fasting.

5 Pounds in One Day!

One pound of fatty tissue is the caloric equivalent of approximately 3500 calories. To burn off this one pound of fat, you would have to eat 500 less calories per day for a week. This, many people find hard to do, consistently. That's for one pound!

But when you fast, you will not find it unusual to lose five pounds the first day and up to 10 pounds in two days!

Now, if you go back to your old eating habits, after a 24-hour or prolonged fast, you will gain the weight back quickly.

Your doctor can recommend a balanced diet which usually contains:

1. No less than 12-14% protein
2. No more than 30% of fat (but not saturated fats)
3. The balance in carbohydrates (eliminating sugars)

**High in
Protein**

Foods high in protein include:
1. Meat
2. Fish
3. Eggs
4. Milk

**High in
Carbohydrates**

Foods high in carbohydrates include:
1. Milk
2. Beans
3. Lentils
4. Potatoes
5. Banana
6. Whole wheat bread

**Saturated
Fats**

Fats are saturated or unsaturated (with some being polyunsaturated).

Fats that are solid are mostly saturated. Saturated, means to be full or satisfied, referring to the fact that the tiny molecules of these fats do not readily combine with other substances—hence they clog arteries. Examples would be most margarines, butter, and fats from meat and hydrogenated cooking fats.

**Unsaturated
Fats**

Fats that are liquid, with some exceptions, are unsaturated. These are chemically unsatisfied and hence their tiny molecules easily combine with other substances— hence they pass through and do not clog arteries. Examples would be vegetable oils and fish oils. Safflower, sunflower-seed, sesame-seed, soy and peanut oil are good sources to use.

It is hard for the person whose overweight is due to overeating to fast. This is because his fondness for food usually gains the victory over his desire to control his intake.

Consistency Needed

Fasting calls both for consistency and strength of will.

Dr. Otto H.F. Buchinger believes that persons with all types of obesity ". . . not only can but should fast!" He states that the waste products and stores of fat, by fasting, are then broken down, burnt up and eliminated.

Dr. Buchinger, in his fasting clinic in Germany, has found that ". . . almost all forms of chronic articular rheumatism and pains in the joints accompanying the menopause respond with gratitude to the treatment, especially if the patient undergoes it year after year."

How Fast Can I Lose Weight by Fasting?

Reports of those who have fasted for a week indicate that one can lose up to 20 pounds in that time period.

In a fast of 4 weeks, one can lost as much as 20% of his original weight.

Dr. Allan Cott reports that British doctors are now using fasting for weight control.

And at Glasgow's Ruchill Hospital, researchers believe that:

> *Total fasting is the most efficient method of reducing weight in obese patients.*

Your most dramatic weight loss comes in the first few days of your fast. After that the rate of weight loss decreases to about a pound or two a day. When fluid has been eliminated from your body by fasting, you begin to live off your fat. Thus the weight loss.

Some Good Advice

In the Bible, the book of Proverbs we read:

> Better is a dish of vegetables
> where love is,
> Than a fattened ox and hatred with it.
> (Proverbs 15:17)

It is not only important for your health what you eat but also how you eat.

Just a moment, take a look at your own home at dinner time. Do you take a minute to say grace and thank the Lord that there is food on the table. Saying grace will set the pace and mood for the entire meal.

And are there any arguments that carry over to the dinner table. Do you harbor a grudge against someone with whom you are eating?

And this rule is very important!!

NEVER, NEVER, NEVER
use the meal time to get into a heated
discussion or display of temper.

Eat slowly. Eat sensibly. But never eat until you are satisfied! Eating till you are full means you have eaten too much!

Then, don't plunge immediately into work. Relax for an half hour by taking a leisurely walk.

Putter a little bit in your garden.

And, if you don't have a garden . . . come over and see mine . . .

and

my parsley!

10

WILL FASTING LOWER MY BLOOD PRESSURE ?

The doctors call it hypertension. You and I know it as high blood pressure.

Hypertension is a condition in which one has a higher blood pressure than judged to be normal.

A Symptom . . .
Not a
Disease

Hypertension is not a disease . . . it is a symptom and its importance depends on the significance of its cause!

<u>Organic</u> hypertension is often due to diseases of the:

1. Heart and arteries
   (atherosclerosis, arteriosclerosis)[1]
2. Kidneys
   (glomerulonephritis)
3. Internal secretory glands

<u>Organic</u> hypertension is mostly acquired. Organic hypertension tends to progress . . . sometimes slow, sometimes quite rapidly. As the progress becomes more acute, it

---

[1] Atherosclerosis: A form of arteriosclerosis in which there are localized ac-<u>cumulations</u> of lipid-containing material within or beneath the inner coat of blood vessels.

Arteriosclerosis: A condition in which there is a <u>thickening</u>, hardening, and loss of elasticity <u>of the walls</u> of blood vessels, especially arteries.

may strike a "target organ." It may strike the cerebral blood vessels, causing a stroke. It may hit the coronaries, causing a heart attack (myocardial infarction). It may effect the kidneys, causing uremia, or your eyes, causing blindness.

Drugs May Produce Adverse Effects

Most physicians try to use the least toxic drugs for mild hypertension. The Medical Letter on Drugs and Therapeutics, a non-profit publication for doctors, states on page 23 of its January, 1975 issue:

All antihypertensive drugs can cause severe adverse effects.

On page 24 of the same newsletter:

Reserpine and other rauwolfia alkaloids deplete tissue of stores of catecholamines[1] and 5-hydroxytryptamine (serotonin), including those in the central nervous system.

Their most disturbing adverse effect is psychic depression that can lead to suicide.

A history of depression is an absolute contraindication to use of rauwolfia alkaloids, but severe depression can also occur in patients without such a history when they take these drugs.

An increased incidence of breast cancer has been reported in patients treated with reserpine (Lancet, 2:669, 672, 675, 1974), although a cause-and-effect relationship has not been established.

---

[1] Catecholamines: Biologically active amines, epinephrine and norepinephrine, derived from the amino acid tyrosine. They have a marked effect on the nervous and cardiovascular systems, metabolic rate, temperature, and smooth muscle.

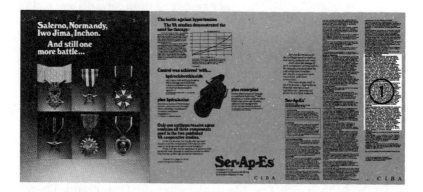

ADVERSE REACTIONS

Reserpine: *Gastrointestinal*—hypersecretion; nausea; vomiting; anorexia; diarrhea. *Cardiovascular*—angina-like symptoms; arrhythmias (particularly when used concurrently with digitalis or quinidine); bradycardia. *Central Nervous System*—drowsiness; depression; nervousness; paradoxical anxiety; nightmares; rare parkinsonian syndrome and other extrapyramidal tract symptoms; CNS sensitization (manifested by dull sensorium, deafness, glaucoma, uveitis, and optic atrophy). *Miscellaneous*—frequently nasal congestion; pruritus; rash; dryness of mouth; dizziness; headache; dyspnea; syncope; epistaxis; purpura and other hematological reactions; impotence or decreased libido; dysuria; muscular aches; conjunctival injection; weight gain; breast engorgement; pseudolactation; gynecomastia; rarely water retention with edema in hypertensive patients.

Hydralazine: *Common*—headache; palpitations; anorexia; nausea; vomiting; diarrhea; tachycardia; angina pectoris. *Less frequent*—nasal congestion; flushing; lacrimation; conjunctivitis; peripheral neuritis, evidenced by paresthesias, numbness, and tingling; edema; dizziness; tremors; muscle cramps; psychotic reactions characterized by depression, disorientation, or anxiety; hypersensitivity (including rash, urticaria, pruritus, fever, chills, arthralgia, eosinophilia, and, rarely, hepatitis); constipation; difficulty in micturition; dyspnea; paralytic ileus; lymphadenopathy; splenomegaly; blood dyscrasias, consisting of reduction in hemoglobin and red cell count, leukopenia, agranulocytosis, and purpura; hypotension; paradoxical pressor response.

Hydrochlorothiazide: *Gastrointestinal*—anorexia, gastric irritation, nausea, vomiting, cramping, diarrhea, constipation, jaundice (intrahepatic cholestatic), pancreatitis. *Central Nervous System*—dizziness, vertigo, paresthesias, headache, xanthopsia. *Dermatologic-Hypersensitivity*—purpura, photosensitivity, rash, urticaria, necrotizing angiitis, Stevens-Johnson syndrome, and other hypersensitivity reactions. *Hematologic*—leukopenia, agranulocytosis, thrombocytopenia, aplastic anemia. *Cardiovascular*—orthostatic hypotension may occur and may be potentiated by alcohol, barbiturates, or narcotics. *Other*—hyperglycemia, glycosuria, hyperuricemia, muscle spasm, weakness, restlessness. Whenever adverse reactions are moderate or severe, reduce dosage or withdraw therapy.

It might be pointed out that The Medical Letter on Drugs and Therapeutics is an independent non-profit publication which provides unbiased critical evaluations of drugs in terms of their effectiveness, adverse effects, and possible alternative medications.

For treatment The Medical Letter continues, in part, on page 25:

> *Drug treatment should start with a thiazide-type diuretic; if this does not produce an adequate response, a second drug may be needed.*

From the previous quotations it should be observed that no drug is really entirely safe or completely adequate in the treating of high blood pressure.

And, if fasting can produce promising results, under your physician's supervision, it certainly should be seriously considered.

We Live in a STRESS Environment

We are living in an age of STRESS! Advertisers on television have conditioned most people that they simply cannot live or enjoy life without their product. **Therefore the grand race begins of trying to earn enough money to buy "just one more thing."**

Then, on the other hand, ravaging inflation sometimes makes it necessary for one to hold two jobs just to be able to feed his family and provide them with essential clothes and pay the mortgage.

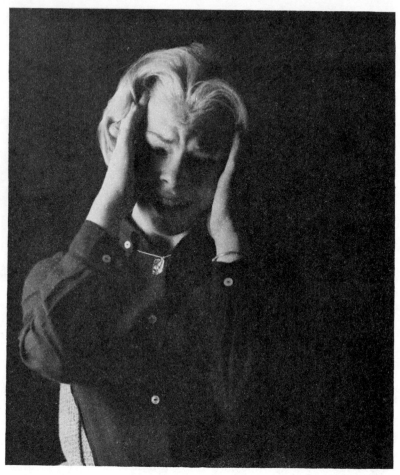

Doctors at the Headache Clinic in New York estimate that nearly 90% of Americans have headaches at one time or another. More than half the visits to doctors' offices each year are for this problem. In the U.S. alone more than $105 million worth of aspirin tablets are consumed each year. Many have reported freedom from headaches after short, periodic, 24-hour fasts. Sufferers of migraine headaches have reported complete relief after medically-supervised fasts of ten days to three weeks.

And to this add the "quickie" meals at fast-food fare drive-ins . . . with their fat-saturated hamburgers and heart-attack inducing french fries.

And what do you come up with?

STRESS!

And what can stress lead to?

HIGH BLOOD PRESSURE plus a myriad other ills!

Warning Signs

So to stay fresh and awake . . . when we get run-down, we gulp a cup of coffee.

Soon we notice warning signs of improper living:

1. Frequent headaches
2. Inner discontent
3. Restlessness
4. Weak concentration
5. Mild agitation
6. Loss of sense of humor

Work, which previously satisfied us now becomes a painful burden.

In the second stage, we notice anxious sensations of heart pain and nervous outbreaks of perspiring.

At the third stage we discover we have high blood pressure or suffer a stroke, a nervous breakdown or experience a heart attack.

When it reaches this point, the breakdown in our health may be so severe that a complete recovery is not possible.

Medical Tribune

and Medical News —

Vol. 16, No. 31 — *world news of medicine and its practice—fast, accurate.* Wednesday, September 3, 1975

McDonald's Corp. May Stop Salting Its French Fries

By MICHAEL HERRING
Medical Tribune Staff

NEW YORK—After an unusual meeting here with members of the Manhattan Central Medical Society and the N.A.A.C.P.'s health care committee, McDonald's Corporation executives are now researching a possible change in the current policy of presalting the french fries served in their franchises, according to Dennis Detzel, manager of corporate responsibility.

Dr. Charles Brown, a psychiatrist who heads the medical society as well as the health care committee, told MEDICAL TRIBUNE he arranged the meeting at Harlem Hospital to increase community awareness of "the kinds of things that people put into their bodies," and, specifically, to find out why McDonald's automatically douses its french fries with salt, a major dietary factor in hypertension.

Problem to Be Studied

The answer Mr. Detzel gave at the meeting was very simple: Because that's the way people want them. Kenneth Clement, dean of the company's "Hamburger University," added that McDonald's salts the fries just enough so that customers won't ask for the more expensive packaged salt.

"The meeting with Dr. Brown really called my attention to the problem of salt as a factor in hypertension," Mr. Detzel said. "It was the first I'd heard that salt could be harmful, but I've already asked Stanford Research Institute to investigate the problem."

Mr. Detzel said he wants to find out whether the salt content of the McDonald's diet is high, middle, or low, and how much salt a person is likely to ingest if he eats three meals a day beneath the golden arches.

Dr. Muriel Petioni, assistant visiting physician at Harlem Hospital and a member of the group that met with Dr. Brown, stressed the importance of calling public attention to the threat of hypertension, especially among blacks.

People Unaware

"High blood pressure and heart disease are much more prevalent among blacks, occur at a much earlier age, and the death rate is higher. The trouble with hypertension is that people usually are unaware of it in its early stages," she said.

An Ounce of Prevention

The purpose of this book is primarily to point out the advantages of fasting . . . but also to make you aware of proper health maintenance <u>before</u> an irreversible illness occurs. I need not remnd you that "an ounce of prevention is worth a pound of cure!"

But I'll remind you anyway!

An ounce of prevention

IS (there is no doubt about it)

worth

a pound of cure!

In hypertension — high blood pressure — a variety of factors from malfunction to nervous strain may combine to create a resistance to the flow of blood through the arterioles, causing the heart to pump harder to surmount this obstacle.

How's Your Arterial Resiliency?

Arterioles are minute arteries. The heart of a man with hypertension may fill half his chest cavity.

In arterial disease the arteries lose their resiliency, the walls harden as a result of the deposit of fatty materials and calcium.

Healthy arterial walls, however, stretch and rebound with each heartbeat.

Fasting aids in the purification of these arteries. Toxics are flushed out of the body, unneeded fat is "burned up" and excreted. One starts to feel young again, there is a lightness in the body, an alertness in the mind.

Fasting, combined with sensible eating habits, are beneficial in the lowering of one's blood pressure.

The arteries of the heart are small. The largest arteries in the heart are no wider than a thin soda straw.

There is much truth in the saying:

You are as old as your arteries.

**Fasting
is
Scriptural**

Fasting is mentioned 74 times in the Bible. You must remember that fasting is not a cure of any disease or ailment. Fasting helps the body help itself. Fasting gives the body a complete rest from the digestive processes so the organs of the body can devote their energies to self-healing and self-rejuvenation.

And fasting can be a definite benefit to those with high blood pressure.

Perhaps we should follow the advice of Jesus, after the disciples came to him and told him of John the Baptist's untimely death at the hands of Herod.

Jesus, upon hearing this sad news, said to his disciples:

*Come ye yourselves apart
into a desert place
and rest a while . . .*

(Mark 6:31)

What good advice for each of us to follow.

In this frenzied pace of today's living it is very easy for one to develop high blood pressure.

We have to learn how to relax and eat properly.

And fasting places us in an aura of relaxation, makes us more aware of nature around us and gives us an opportunity not only to rest our mind but also our body.

And by so doing, our life suddenly takes on a new purpose and meaning.

11

HOW DO I BEGIN FASTING?

Primitive people thought of their medicine men at least as highly as we enlightened people think of our men of medicine. Indeed, they were regarded not merely as physicians, but they were regarded as holy men as well.

No doubt, more of today's physicians would have even greater success if they were on a talking basis with Jesus Christ, the Great Physician.

Primitive societies often believe that spirits are responsible for the rain, the heat and the sun as well as for serious illnesses.

To get rid of an illness, an Eskimo goes into a trance, takes a "trip" to the supernatural world and returns to this one with a "cure."

Witch Doctors Frighten Disease

The African witch doctor tries to frighten the disease. He chases an evil spirit by biting, beating, punching, kicking or even stamping the patient.

If the patient survives this drastic therapy, the witch doctor attempts to lure the spirit away to take up residence in an animal.

Do our modern medical men follow the same technique? Not quite. Instead of stomping on us . . . we are subjected to long waits in a waiting room . . . where we study the office wallpaper or read magazines published during the Civil War.

When a patient goes to an African witch doctor, he really believes his stomping and screaming will cure him.

And there are three distinct factors that a physician uses to his benefit which are similar to that of the African witch doctor.

The Doctor's Helpers

The <u>first</u> factor the doctor relies on is <u>psychological.</u>

How many times have you felt sick . . . but just to get to that waiting room and see the doctor provides for you a great comfort. Many illnesses are intensified or generated by anxiety, loneliness or depression.

The <u>second</u> factor on which physicians rely is the fact that at least three-quarters of the diseases that affect people are in time overcome by the body's own action! And this occurs, whether or not it is assisted by the doctor's remedies! <u>Nature is its own healer!</u>

The <u>third</u> reason for a doctor's success: <u>his knowledge of effective remedies.</u> And here, doctors deserve great credit!

Illness Costs Sky Rocket!

Have you ever taken a moment to figure just how much money and time you have spent on doctor's visits? And in hospitals. Just for fun, figure out in dollars and cents what you spent in medical bills this past

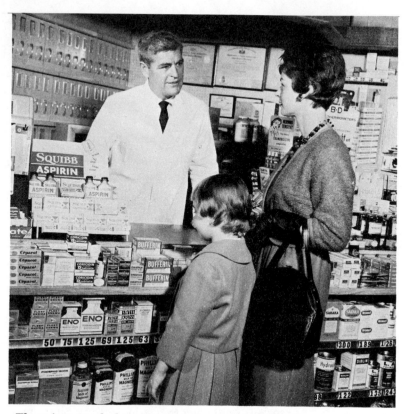

There is no such thing as a safe drug! Dr. Henry Simmons, formerly chief of drugs at the U.S. Food and Drug Administration (FDA) has stated: *"You can't have an effective drug that also doesn't have the potential of hurting somebody . . . a completely safe drug is not only unrealistic but unattainable. . . ."*

Americans spend over $8 billion each year on legal drugs — $3.6 billion of it for over-the-counter preparations such as headache pills, cold remedies and tonics. The average American visits the doctor's office three times a year. Many would be insulted if a doctor prescribed organic vitamin supplements or periodic fasting. Patients usually expect a prescription when they visit a doctor. That little white piece of paper is their security blanket. And the drug that prescription makes possible, they believe, is the cure-all for all their problems . . . when, in reality . . . **it could be the beginning of their problems!**

year and include headache and cold remedies you purchased in the drug store, too.

Now, to that add the cost of one day's meals each week throughout the year — (3 per day X 52 weeks) 156 meals!

Then, determine that right now . . . beginning this week, you will fast one day a week. At the end of the year, see how much money you save, how few headaches and colds you suffer and how much more time you have on your hands.

How to Save Time and Money!

For in fasting one day each week you will save the cost of 156 meals (which you don't need) but you will also add approximately 156 hours to your time availability to do other things . . . or about 6 additional days!

And — in my opinion — you will feel better, more alert, have a happier marriage, look and feel younger, slow down your aging process, lose weight and save money!

Psychosomatic Illnesses

The scientific physician realizes that a large proportion of illnesses are psychosomatic; that is resulting from the mind's effect on the body. This is why, incidentally, healing evangelists are so successful. They get people to get their mind off themselves and their problems and place them in the hands of God. Unfortunately, some healing evangelists use this to achieve their own selfish aims. And people pay the evangelist through their offerings.

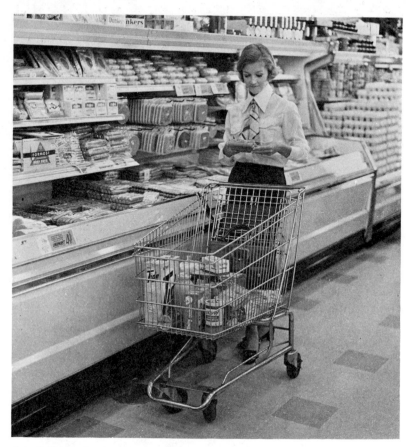

It's difficult for the housewife to buy wholesome foods without additives. Pre-packaged cold cuts and hot dogs, as an example, are loaded with preservatives such as sodium nitrite and nitrate. Packaged cheeses are preserved with disodium phosphate. One hot dog has as much as 533 mg. of sodium. One ounce of American processed cheese has 440 mg. of sodium. Many foods are loaded with salt. Salt is sodium-chloride. The best-known malady suspected to be due to salt is high blood pressure. An estimated 25 million Americans have high blood pressure! Recently, it has been revealed that even the plastic used to package cold cuts contains chemicals harmful to the body.

The doctor uses the same technique, sometimes even in special cases giving pills that have no physical value at all, called placebos. And you get better. And you pay the doctor through his fee.

Now fasting, will give your body a complete rest. Through this rest and period of rejuvenation, your mind and your senses will become keener and more alert.

And this very process . . . as in psychosomatic healing . . . may also effect a healing in your life.

Those Who Should Not Fast

Before you consider fasting you should realize that there are those who should never fast.[1] If you have:

1. Bleeding ulcers
2. Cancer
3. Diabetes (juvenile)
4. Gout
5. Liver diseases
6. Kidney diseases
7. A recent heart attack
8. Cerebral diseases
9. Tumors

Children and young people should never fast without their doctor's approval. Children can safely fast one day a week if their protein intake on all the other days of that week exceeds the minimum requirement.

Therefore, before you fast, consult your

---

[1]Some fasting clinics would not agree to this statement. In their own experiences with the conducting of thousands of fasts, they have found beneficial results even with those suffering some of the illnesses listed. It's always best to check with a competent physician whom you trust.

physician. He is the best judge of your tolerance to fasting because he knows your health condition. This is a rule everyone should follow.

Now, as with vitamin supplements, your doctor may laugh at you when you suggest fasting but approve it for one day per week saying, "Well, it certainly can't hurt you."

But for your own best interests, be sure to consult your physician.

Therefore, the first step to fasting is:

1. Secure your doctor's permission.

The second step to fasting is:

2. Approach it with a positive outlook.

Don't go into a fasting program with the negative idea, "Well, I don't believe it, but I'll try it."

Remember, the first step on the road to healing for the native who went to the African witch doctor and to the patient that goes to the medical doctor, is BELIEVING that such action will bring a recovery.

So, BE OPTIMISTIC! Wipe the doubts from the cobwebs of your mind.

Fasting Works

Fasting is not new. It is mentioned 74 times in the Bible. Multiple thousands of people have fasted before you and they have found IT WORKS.

Believing in the laws of nature, follow the viewpoint that fasting is a logical way to restore more vibrant body function. And exercise CONFIDENCE!

The third step to fasting is:

3. Don't give up!

Fasting is a good preventive measure against illness and it can also be curative therapy.

But if you have been accustomed to eating "3 square meals a day" for 20, 30 or 50 years, it may prove difficult at first to skip one meal, two meals, three meals.

How to Succeed in Fasting

It may take real willpower. And remember, when you fast, and your willpower starts to weaken . . . strengthen it by saying:

I am flushing out the poisons
   from my system.
I am slowing down my aging process.
I am getting rid of sick headaches.
I am flushing out constipation.
I am going to war against fatigue.
I will feel better and brighter!
Don't be a failure in fasting!

A fool often fails because he thinks what is difficult is easy, and a wise man because he thinks what is easy is difficult!

And when you are on your fast, and you see the rest of your family eating a succulent steak dinner, just remember the wisdom of the old Southern preacher who said:

> When you're looking at your neighbor's
> melon patch,
> brother, you can't keep your mouth
>   from watering,
> but you can run!

Through willpower and determination, you will find yourself well on the way to successful fasting.

12

THE 24-HOUR FAST

Most people have found out that short fasts will achieve as great or greater benefits than long fasts.

Paul C. Bragg, who has been supervising fasts for over 50 years, himself fasts

1 24-hour period each week
2 7-10 day fasts each year

He eats two meals a day; the first one at noon.

He wrote his book, The Miracle of Fasting, at 85 years of age. He states that as a result of fasting periodically all his life:

> ... I pride myself on having the
> most flexible joints of any man,
> regardless of age.
> I perform difficult yoga postures
> with ease while standing on my head.
> I am a human dynamo.
> I get more out of living in one day
> than the average person gets out
> of five.
> I have an unlimited amount of
> energy for work and play!
> I never get tired ... sleepy – yes
> ... but never do I get that
> worn-out, exhausted feeling.[1]

In this book, we are recommending

---

[1]Paul C. Bragg, The Miracle of Fasting, (Santa Ana: Health Science), 1974, pp. 35, 61.

primarily the 24-hour fast. There are longer fast periods. Some people fast 3-7 days at a time. In fasting clinics longer fasts of 20-30 days are not unusual. Very rarely, however, is a fast extended beyond this time.

**Fasting
is not
Starving**

Fasting is not starving. Fasting is going without food for a stated period. Your energy requirements of body metabolism during fasting are supplied by the oxidization of fats. Fasting ends when the forces of starvation begin.

Dr. Allan Cott, in his book, Fasting: The Ultimate Diet, gives an excellent definition of the difference between fasting and starving on page 56:

> *A person is fasting
> as long as he continues
> to eat nothing
> and experiences no real hunger.
> Starvation begins
> when the body has consumed its
> spare resources,
> craves food, and –
> for whatever reason –
> continues to be deprived of food.*

**Your Body
Will Signal You**

Dr. Cott, as well as others, believe it takes a long fast to cross the line into starvation. The body will signal you when its time to break a long fast. And that does not usually occur until at least the 25th day.

Long periods of fasting, those over 5-7 days, are generally conducted in a fasting clinic under proper medical supervision.

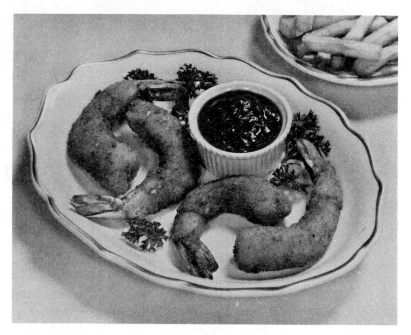

Look at this plate. The only thing nutritionally of real value to your body is the parsley. And yet, that's the one thing most people simply shove aside as just "decorative material." Just 3 ounces of french fried shrimp has 190 calories and 158 mg. of sodium and is loaded with cholesterol.

And 10 french fried potatoes have 140 calories and they are usually doused with salt, a major dietary factor in high blood pressure! French fries are one of the worst foods you can eat. Because, in the frying process, the composition of frying oil is changed, making much of it virtually impossible to assimilate into your blood stream. Instead, it builds up as plaques on your arterial walls and is a major cause of heart attacks and strokes.

Next time you order a meal of fried shrimp and french fried potatoes . . . give them to your worst enemy and you eat the parsley! You'll be healthier for it!

When Should
I Begin
My Fast

A 24-hour fast, in my opinion, is best begun after breakfast. Skip lunch and dinner and breakfast of the following day. And go off your fast with dinner.

Paul Bragg does not believe in eating breakfast. He has two meals a day. You may find two meals a day . . . lunch and dinner, beneficial for you, too. There is much merit to this.

But at any rate . . . begin your fast by abstaining from lunch.

And do NOT put one piece of food in your mouth until the next day at lunch in the early afternoon. In otherwords, make sure you go without FOOD for 24 hours.

Paul Bragg often, on his one-day-a-week fast goes for 36 hours without food. After a few one-day fasts of 24 hour periods you may wish to switch to a 36-hour period without food . . . each week.

Drink
Only
Water

During your fast . . . eat no food. Eat no fruits. Eat no vegetables. Do not take vitamin pills. Do not chew gum. Do not eat candy. And certainly, do not smoke!

Do not drink milk. Do not drink juices.

During a fast, the only thing you take is WATER!

There is no limit to the amount of water you can drink, within reason. But you should drink at least two quarts of water each day you fast. Water helps flush your body of the impurities. It keeps your body from becoming dehydrated. And it relieves the "hunger pangs" you may experience.

Distilled vs. Mineral Water

There are two schools of thought on what kind of water to drink. Some, like Paul Bragg, believe you should only drink

distilled water

Dr. Cott and others believe you should drink

mineral water

In either case, I would **not** recommend the tap water from your own faucet as the best choice.

My wife, Mary and I drink distilled water during our 24-hour fasts.

And to make it more pleasing to the taste we follow Paul Bragg's recommendation of adding to a glass of distilled water:

½ teaspoon of honey
½ teaspoon of lemon

We have found this to be very satisfactory.

But Won't I Feel Hungry?

This may be difficult for you to believe. But going without food for one day, for two days, or for 10 or more days . . . you will NOT feel hungry. Generally by the 25th day of a fast, hunger pains begin. This is a clear indication that the fast should be stopped.

But we are talking about the 24-hour fast.

You will NOT feel hungry. The moment you do get "hunger pains" you take a glass of water. And immediately those hunger pains will disappear.

After all, you have trained your stomach to expect food at regular intervals three times

How Fasting May Affect You • 153

a day.

You can't "untrain" it overnight.

But by drinking the water, that hunger feeling in your stomach will quickly disappear.

What to Expect

Now if you are a coffee or tea drinker or take alcoholic beverages you will get a dull headache. Why? Because you have conditioned your body to a regular stimulant. When you take this unhealthy stimulant away you will get a reaction. During your 24-hour fast your body is going to begin the process of flushing out these old buried residues of poisons.

The headache or sluggish feeling you may experience is an indication that the fast is WORKING by beginning the process of eliminating the poisons that have been accumulating in your body.

A woman executive in New York gives this report of her fasting experience:

> Two weeks without food is the standard stretch, [at the Buchinger Clinic in Germany] and it is – surprisingly enough – painless.
> When one stops eating, appetite vanishes. It was no problem to pass right by those tempting pastry shops in the nearby village and to limit myself to mineral water.[1]

My Personal Experience

I, too, honestly felt before I began my first 24-hour fast that I would be very hungry when fasting. I know that in my normal,

---

[1]Alan Cott, M.D., Fasting: The Ultimate Diet (New York: Bantam Books, Inc.), 1975, p. 66.

everyday life, if I go without eating at too long an interval I get hunger pains.

Perhaps you may even feel weak when you are delayed in eating a meal.

But I was surprised to discover that in fasting, I experienced no real hunger pains. Those gentle reminders that it was time to eat were quickly alleviated the moment I drank my glass of water.

And that glass of water carried me for another 3 hours very adequately.

You should drink at least 2 quarts of water each day you fast.

So believe the advice of those who have and who are fasting . . .

YOU WILL NOT FEEL HUNGRY!

One thing you will notice, however, you will suddenly find about 2½ to 3 extra hours on your hands . . . because that would be the time you normally spend eating. At first, you may not know what to do with this extra time. But, if you're industrious, you'll be able to use the time wisely taking care of all those odds and ends that you never had time for before.

Or, and this may be difficult for you to do, just pick up a good book and

RELAX

out in the fresh air or on your sun porch. Learn the art of taking it easy both mentally and physically.

Take a few moments to study nature and the beauty of the trees and flowers around you. I have a morning glory vine I trained to twine up a tree. And each morning as its delicate pale blue blossoms open up . . . I discover anew the real meaning of creation.

And with the extra time on your hands . . . if your family is also fasting, you will find extra money in your pocket!

This is one pleasant side benefit of fasting which I am sure you will not find distressing!

After my fast, I found that my appetite was sharp and greatly enhanced **but I did not have to eat as much food at each meal to be satisfied.** My hay fever, which bothers me in late August, simply vanished! My weight dropped from 150 to 145 (I'm 5' 10"). I feel 100% better and more alert. It is surprising how I get new ideas for books that normally just didn't come as quickly prior to fasting 1 day a week. I started with 24-hour fasts once a week. Now I take a 36-hour fast weekly and find this, in my particular case, the more productive for me personally.

Who knows! In just 24 hours, you can be a bright NEW PERSON!

13

HOW TO BREAK THE 24-HOUR FAST

Well, your fast is about to end . . . and you keep telling yourself:

I can hardly wait. Boy, am I going to plow into a nice, thick, juicy steak. And with all the trimmings, too!

And that's exactly the wrong thing to do!

Whether, in your fast, you experienced any minor discomfort or not . . . the purification of your system was in operation.

Perhaps you will have a headache, a little gnawing in the stomach.

You may notice that your tongue becomes coated. This is a good sign. For your tongue is the "mirror" of your body. It will reflect the amount of waste matter that is being eliminated from your system.

And if you fast for more than a day, this coating becomes even more evident. It may be thick and white.

But this is a good sign. For it is evidence to you of the toxic wastes that have been fermenting within your body system.

**Inside your
Intestines**

Your intestines are about 24 feet long, and are divided into the small intestine and large intestine or colon.

According to Taber's Cyclopedic Medical Dictionary, 12th Edition, the total surface of the small intestine is about 8,611 square feet! The small intestine is greatly enlarged by means of (a) numerous folds and (b) finger-like projections called villi.

What you eat starts at your mouth and passes through 30 feet of alimentary canal which ends at the anus.

The nutritious food you eat, in this process, benefits your body and also aids in regular elimination.

The junk foods you eat, must also pass through this 30 feet of "tubing" but much of the residue of the poisons lodge in various places in your system and eventually you end up ill and with bowel problems.

**When the
Villi
Become
Villains**

The small intestine presents one of the many mysteries of nutrition. It is here that most of the nutrients in the food are absorbed by the body.

The villi, fingerlike tentacles that line the inner walls, look like the pile of a carpet. And it is these villi which are the instruments of the absorption process.

**3500 Villi
Per
Square Inch**

These sensitive villi are about 1/25th of an inch long. And a square inch of intestine holds about 3500 of these densely packed villi.

The villi are your friends as long as you treat them right. But start loading them up with too many:

1. Starches and sugars
2. Fat, grease and fried foods
3. Foods loaded with additives

and they will let you know about it in no uncertain terms. And the villi will become villains because of your mistreatment.

This may be in the form of colicky, sharp abdominal pains, distention of the abdomen, nausea and vomiting, a change in appearance of the stool, loss of weight, blood in the stool.

The doctors may call your problem:

1. Mesenteric Vascular Occlusion
2. Intussusception
3. Acute Organic Intestinal Obstruction
4. Sprue Syndrome
5. Chronic Nonspecific Ulcerative Colitis
6. Diverticulosis & Diverticulitis
7. Polyps

But whatever big name they use to call it, it could be as a result of your bad eating habits.

Back to the Tongue

So, when you see your tongue become coated during a fast, remember it is a good sign. Also remember that your tongue is a mirror of your intestines! And the junk that accumulates on your tongue is only an indication of the junk you have been accumulating in your body. It is the tip of the iceberg!

This evidence in itself should convince you that you should give your body a weekly housecleaning by 24-hour fasts, with your physician's approval.

A Coated Tongue

When your tongue coats up, brush it with a soft toothbrush to get off the accumulated toxic waste. Rinse your mouth with warm water.

Once your fast is over you should notice a difference in your tongue.

On longer fasts the natural disappearance of the coating on the tongue is an indication that it is time to break your fast.

But on 24-hour fasts a complete cleansing is not possible. However, on each repeated 24-hour fast, you will notice more and more improvement as your body rids itself of the poisons that you have accumulated over the years through food mismanagement.

How to Break Your Fast

Have you ever thought what you call your morning meal?

Break
Fast

That is where the word originates. You have been without food all night. And in the morning, when you arise you break this fast by having breakfast.

While children should have a good breakfast, to sustain them through the early school hours ... adults may not find this necessary.

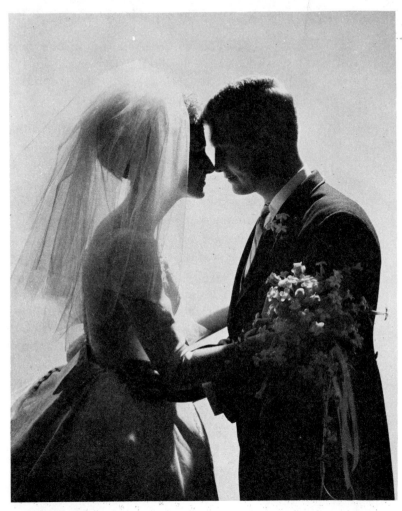

Remember the spark and vitality you had in the first few weeks of married life? Fasting, one day a week, every week, can renew that harmony of love!

Paul Bragg, as mentioned before, does not believe in having a breakfast. He believes that the body must earn its food through exercise. And that loading the digestive system with breakfast is not beneficial. I would tend to agree with him. A drink of distilled water with a half teaspoon of honey and lemon will satisfy your hunger pangs. And this MINI-FAST daily may provide you with energy and alertness you may have never experienced before.

But this is important.

Ease off Fast Gradually

Never, never, never load up your stomach with a heavy meal immediately after breaking your fast.

Your First Meal

The very first food to reach your stomach after a 24-hour fast should be:

a raw vegetable salad

And don't pour commercial salad dressings on it!

Get some fresh carrots and cabbage and grate them. Cut up some red-ripe tomatoes, celery and lettuce or watercress.

And don't forget the parsley!

Then take a fresh lemon or orange and squeeze the juice of this fruit over your salad. **Also . . .**

Use no salt.

The Day Your Tastebuds Come Alive!

And you'll be amazed how delicious this first meal will taste. Suddenly you will discover that your taste buds have become alive.

Over the years you deadened your taste-buds by pouring all sorts of poisonous additives and improper food down your 30 foot canal. Part of these poisons, perhaps unknown to you, ended up coating your tastebuds and deadening them.

Have you ever seen an accoustical ceiling — you know those square panels in the ceiling with tiny holes in them?

Let's Look At Your Tastebuds

Imagine your tongue as an accoustical ceiling. Imagine the thousands of holes in this ceiling. Now, your tongue picks up four primary sensations of taste: sweet, bitter, sour (or acid), and salt.

The four types of taste receptors are located in taste buds which are mainly on the front, back and sides of the tongue's upper surface. Sweetness and saltiness predominate at the tongue's tip. Sourness predominates at the sides. Bitterness at the back.

The center of the tongue is virtually without the ability to taste. While not all taste buds are on the tongue, the primary ones are. You have about 3000 taste buds.

Now, if year after year, you kept putting a new coat of paint over that accoustical ceiling in your church . . . soon the efficiency of that ceiling would be diminished. From a distance it may look the same, but a close-up inspection would show that the tiny perforated holes were beginning to clog up. It would no longer absorb sound efficiently.

Your tongue acts much in the same way. Year after year you keep pouring

**Do You
Realize
What
You Are Doing?**

> parahydroxybenzoates
> calcium propionate
> butylated hydroxyanisole
> ethylene-diamine tetraacetic acid
> nitrite
> nitrate
> methyl anthranilate

and four pounds of other junk into your body . . . the Temple of the Holy Spirit . . . and you start belching, experience flatulence, constipation, heartburn and your villi become villains.

And your taste buds, poisoned by your reckless eating habits, soon lose their sensitivity. You can no longer define those delicate tastes that once gave you great satisfaction.

And as age progresses you may lose nearly all sense of taste.

You may have simply clogged up your taste buds . . . much like the painted up accoustical ceiling tile.

**Why Did
I Say
All That?**

I said all that to say this . . . when you break your fast . . . start with a raw salad.

And notice how your taste buds, perhaps for the first time in years, suddenly come alive as you crunch down on the juicy cabbage and crackle through those raw car-

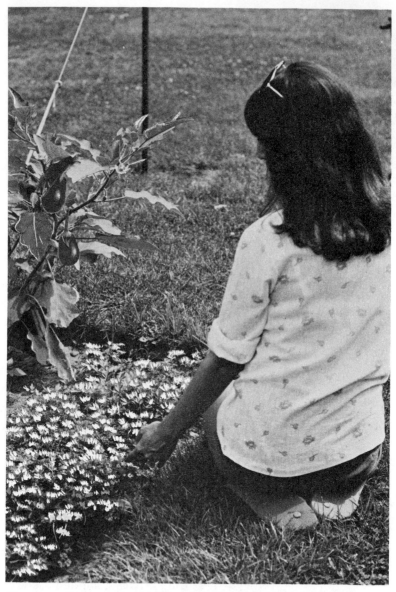

Daughter, Doreen, who is also my excellent proofreader, surveys our bountiful crop of parsley. And that's our eggplant to the left. Have you ever planted eggplant? They are fascinating to watch grow!

rots. You will have never realized, perhaps, that carrots had such an exhilirating taste.

Now you may not fall in love with the parsley.

But you'll feel much better.

Forget Animal Products

Never break a fast with the eating of meat or cheese or butter or nuts. And don't drink milk immediately after a fast.

Ease out of your fast slowly. You will discover that, after a fast, it does not take as much food to satisfy your appetite!

Continue to drink water in adequate quantity. A quart of water a day is recommended.

Dr. Allan Cott suggests the mixing of two quarts of water with one quart of orange juice or apricot juice and to drink this mixture slowly throughout the day after breaking the fast.

By having for your first meal a salad with plenty of water you are in effect helping your own housecleaning. The salad roughage plus the water acts as a broom throughout your entire alimentary canal.

Your Second Meal

By the second meal, after a 24-hour fast, you can begin to eat meats or fish and other nutritional foods.

But remember, eat in moderation. Do NOT load your stomach up so you leave the table "stuffed."

By so doing you are negating much of the good you have realized through the fast.

If you have had the willpower to stick through a 24-hour fast, then certainly you can exert that same willpower to eat sensibly.

And then, why not determine that you are going to have your own garden.

Don't tell me, "I can't, I live in an apartment and don't have any ground."

That's no excuse.

Rent a small plot of ground in your community. Or, if you can, start one on the roof of your apartment . . .

Or start a small herb garden on several windowsills.

And, oh yes.

Don't forget to plant parsley!

14

HOW LONG SHOULD I FAST ?

In this book my main emphasis is on a regular weekly fast of 24 hours.

If, with your doctor's consent, after having tried the 24-hour fast for a period of time, you wish to go on a longer fast be sure to keep in touch with your physician.

Many people first start on a 24-hour fast, progress to a 3-day fast and eventually to a 7-10 day fast. For a longer fast of 25-30 days it is best to do so at a fasting clinic where you can be kept under constant medical supervision.

If you go on a 3-day fast, as an example, the rule of thumb is that you should take 3 days to break that fast.

During longer fasts it is advisable to let someone else drive your car. For long periods of fasting can lead to euphoria, a mild elation which may cause you not to be as responsive to necessary quick action when driving.

During a fast of 3 days or more be sure to get plenty of rest and sun, preferably in the morning. A short walk is also beneficial.

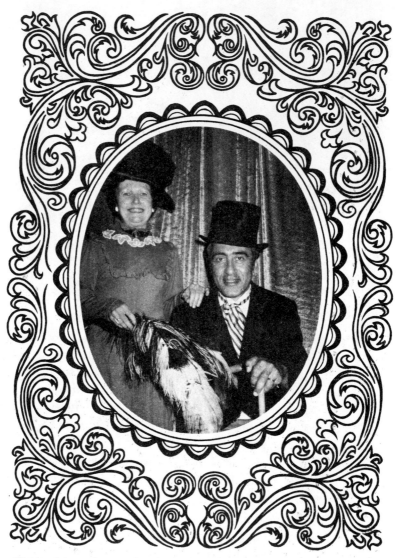

Pictured is author and wife, Mary, in old fashion attire. Photo was taken in Ocean City, New Jersey on boardwalk.

Perhaps it is time we go back to the old fashioned remedies for good health. Let's not rely solely on so-called prescription "miracle drugs" to cure all our ills instantly ... ills that may have been brought about by poor nutritional habits. Remember, there is no such thing as a safe drug!

In longer fasts, however, it is important that you do not deplete your energy.

One Man's Fasting Schedule

Paul Bragg fasts 7-10 days at a time four times a year, along with his weekly fast of 24-36 hours. He finds this very beneficial. You may, too.

His quarterly fasts are: the first part of January, early spring, mid-summer and late October.

Paul Bragg fasts a total of 75 days a year. Such consistent fasting will make your mouth taste sweeter, your breath cleaner and your overall well-being more alive and refreshed.

Elimination Diminishes

In a fast from 3 days to 10 days you may find that your bowels will stop moving. This is normal. After all you are not eating, just drinking water. After you break your fast you should find that your bowels will move more efficiently and regularly.

This is particularly true if you make sure that 50% of the foods that you eat are in their raw, natural state.

Get to start liking salads, bran cereals and other raw foods and fruits.

While writing this book in late August . . . with the exception of the one 24-hour period that I fasted . . . I ate light meals.

A Nutritious Meal

My meals included a generous supply of bean sprouts (which I grew on my kitchen table) salads and occasionally, a parsley sandwich.

A parsley sandwich?

Yes. Try it, it's delicious!

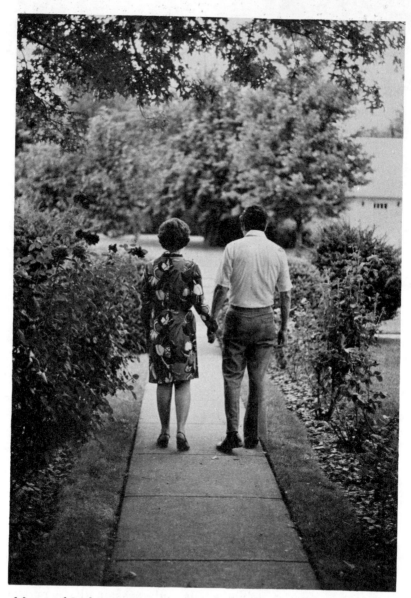

Mary and I take a walk around the block almost every evening. You, too, should enjoy this form of relaxation and exercise away from the cares of the day. Forget about the transient things you consider important business activity and explore the wonders of nature and the vitality of fresh air and exercise.

And here in the library as I type this manuscript, I have by my side a bowl of raw, unsalted almonds and soy beans and some sunflower seeds mixed in.

When I get a hunger signal from my stomach . . . I chew on a few nuts.

The Word is Spreading

First my wife and I decided to fast.

And we feel better for it.

Yesterday, my son-in-law began a 24-hour fast. He drank only distilled water. He noticed pains in his legs. He slept better and he awoke refreshed.

Perhaps even before this book is published others in my family and relatives will take on the benefits derived from fasting.

Who knows!

Put a Spring Back in Your Step

But if I can bring a spring back into your step. If I can for a brief moment help you halt the raging destruction of the aging process. And if I can keep you out of the hospital . . . this book will have been worthwhile!

Fasting is not the end of all your ills.

But fasting could be the beginning of a new and better life.

How long did you sleep last night? Did you toss and turn?

Did you go to bed tired?

And did you wake up also tired?

What about the joints in your body? Are they stiff and sore? Do you feel them creaking every time you move?

Shun Cakes and Creams

How is your appetite? Does it relish all the cakes and creams and candies but shun the carrots and cabbage and cauliflower?

Does your back ache, your head ache and your feet ache?

Is there more gas in your stomach than there is in your car?

Do you feel life has lost its purpose, as far as you are concerned? Do you find goals you set for yourself, unfulfilled, because you just don't have the energy or willpower to carry them out?

Do you find yourself snapping at your wife, your husband and your children?

Turn Duty into Joy

Has love turned into a duty instead of a joy?

Do the promises of God seem to be just empty words?

Do you feel old at 35 or 47 or 87?

Well, there is no reason that you should be!

Would you like to LIVE AGAIN triumphantly? Or are you going to say, "I just know it won't work for me."

If you are tired of being tired . . .
then, dear friend,
for your sake and to
improve your testimony to God
who provided you with a body that is,
if you are a believer, His Holy Temple,
try
FASTING one 24-hour period each week.

Of course, let your family doctor <u>first</u> know of your intentions!

And after the fast,
do me a favor,
and
try eating some parsley!

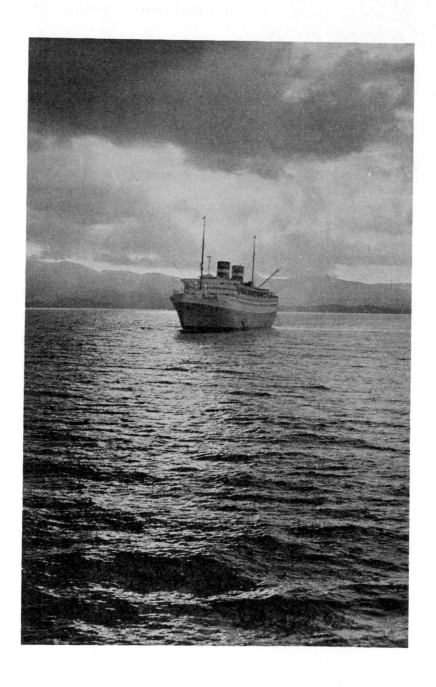

IT'S YOUR LIFE!

It's your life . . .
Given you at birth
    and set out to sail
    on life's sea.

How long your voyage
    depends on you
    and on your crew

If your first mate is sugar
And your deck hands french fries
And your generator, ice cream
And all types of pies

If your fuel pump is whipped
With whiskey and gin
And cigarettes pumping
More smoke within

Your pipes will get rusty
Your voyage cut short
And you'll hear the bad news
In the medical report.

No magic prescription
Will cure all your ills
Nor will the aspirin
Or miracle pills

The sea of adversity
Will sweep o'er your bow
And the engine of life
Will forget you somehow!

But it's your life.
You choose the crew.
For the length of your voyage
WILL DEPEND ON YOU!

                    Salem Kirban

Epilogue

Do you want to know something?

I would love to hear from you . . . personally, after you have completed 4 or 5 weekly fasts of 24-36 hours.

Honestly, it would thrill my heart to have you write me.

Briefly, let me know what beneficial results you experienced during this fast.

If you will, write in this format:

1. Your full name and address
2. Your age (or say, "in the 50's," etc.)
3. Your sex; male or female
4. Date you began fasting
5. How many 24-hour fasts you have taken
6. Side-effects you noticed such as headaches, leg pains, etc.
7. Benefits you noticed after your fast.
   (Spiritual as well as physical benefits)
   Did it improve your home life?
   Did you feel better physically?
      In what way?
   Did it bring you closer to the Lord?

It will be an encouragement to me and who knows, perhaps then I'll write another book on steps to better health!

A SPECIAL NOTE TO DOCTORS

Forgive me if I took a few swipes at the medical profession. I love you! I marvel at your skills. And I would appreciate your taking the time to write me . . . whatever your reaction.

And if you, too, take the 24-hour fasting program once a week, write me and let me know your results. And do me a favor, dear doctor. Please eat parsley!

SALEM KIRBAN
2117 Kent Road, Huntingdon Valley, Pennsylvania 19006 U.S.A.

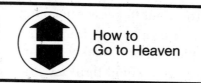

ETERNAL LIFE		How to Go to Heaven

You have just read
HOW TO KEEP HEALTHY and HAPPY by FASTING.

The advice given in this book, we hope, will make it possible for you to live a long life in good health.

But I would not be fulfilling my obligation to you if all I told you was how to be better physically. For our life span on this earth rarely exceeds 100 years.

And, more important, is your spiritual welfare. You may be in the best of health physically, but suffer from a cancer of the soul that will follow you through an eternity.

You can have life eternal by accepting Jesus Christ as your personal Saviour, your Messiah and Lord.

Are you going to continue to place your faith in man and his abilities to surmount any problem you may have? We have polluted our earth already beyond saving! Man certainly has not solved his problems in the past and there is no reason to believe he will in the future!

Are you going to say to yourself . . . "this certainly is worth thinking about" . . . and then put it aside and forget about it?

OR

Are you going to face the facts squarely . . . and get your own house in order now . . . while there is still time?

Many people refuse to accept the Bible as the Word of God because of several reasons.

Some say: "The church-going people I know are hypocrites. . . ."

And to an extent, some are. Certainly, however, this points to the fact that all of us have sinned . . . no one is perfect. However, we cannot get to Heaven based on actions of other people (whether good or bad). Our entrance to Heaven is based on our own personal decision to trust Christ as our personal Saviour and Lord.

"Verily, verily, I say unto you, He that heareth my word, and believeth on him that sent me, hath everlasting life, and shall not come into condemnation; but is passed from death unto life. (John 5:24)

Others say: "The churches I know are no different from the world. They are simply social centers with do-gooders."

And to some extent, this is true. For many ministers and their churches have departed from the true ministry of preaching the Gospel.

Now the Spirit speaketh expressly, that in the latter times some shall depart from the faith. . ." (1 Timothy 4:1)

While others say: "I cannot accept the Bible's plan for eternal life, because I cannot scientifically prove that life exists after death . . . a real Heaven . . . a real Hell."

Such people are well prophetically described in 2 Timothy 3:5

"Having a form of godliness, but denying the power thereof: from such turn away."

For Christ did indeed rise from the dead and. . .

". . .He showed himself alive after His passion by many infallible proofs, being seen of them forty days, and speaking of the things pertaining to the kingdom of God."

The main question however is this:

WHAT WILL YOU DO WITH JESUS?

Will you state that He never existed?

Will you simply say He was a good man who did good things?

Will you say His message is not relevant to our enlightened age?

Would you buy a car without first finding out the facts relevant to that car?

Would you invest money in a venture without first finding out details of that organization?

Would you get married without first finding out more about the individual with whom you pledge your entire life?

Your answer would probably be NO to each of these last three questions.

Then WHAT ABOUT JESUS? WHAT ABOUT HEAVEN? WHAT ABOUT HELL? WHAT ABOUT ETERNAL LIFE? WHAT ABOUT ETERNAL DAMNATION? WHAT ABOUT YOUR FUTURE AND THAT OF YOUR CHILDREN?

I am sure you will agree that your life here on earth will not go on and on. Any funeral director can attest to that fact. Any nurse or doctor can tell you that physical life on this earth someday ceases for each of us.

And if you have examined world conditions you will admit that the world is certainly not getting better and better. World leaders and scientists everywhere acknowledge the fact that the next 30 years will give us more complex problems in population growth, in famine, in crime, and in war.

Then what can you do?

Well, you can simply choose to ignore Christ and the Scriptures . . . go on living your life, doing the best you know how to meet your problems, work and provide an income for your family, set aside a nest egg for retirement in a highly questionable future.

But THEN WHAT?

What happens when it comes time for you to depart from this earth?

Then WHAT WILL YOU DO WITH JESUS?

It takes NO DECISION on your part to go to Hell!

It does take a DECISION on your part, however, to go to Heaven!

> He that believeth on Him is not condemned: but he that believeth not is condemned already, because he hath not believed in the name of the only begotten Son of God (John 3:18).

Here are five basic observations in the Bible of which you should be aware:

1. ALL SINNED
> For all have sinned, and come short of the glory of God (Romans 3:23).

2. ALL LOVED
> For God so loved the world, that He gave His only begotten Son, that whosoever believeth in Him should not perish, but have everlasting life (John 3:16).

3. ALL RAISED
> Marvel not at this: for the hour is coming, in which all that are in the graves shall hear his voice,
> And shall come forth; they that have done good, unto the resurrection of life; and they that have done evil, unto the resurrection of damnation (John 5:28, 29).

4. ALL JUDGED
> . . . We shall all stand before the judgment seat of Christ (Romans 14:10).
> And I saw the dead, small and great, stand before God; and the books were opened . . . (Revelation 20:12).

5. ALL BOW
> . . . At the name of Jesus every knee should bow . . . (Philippians 2:10).

Right now, in simple faith, you can have the wonderful assurance of eternal life.

Ask yourself, honestly, the question. . .

WHAT WILL I DO WITH JESUS?

Will you accept Jesus Christ as your personal Saviour and Lord or will you reject Him?

This you must decide yourself. No one else can decide that for you. The basis of your decision should be made on God's Word — the Bible.

God tells us the following:

> ". . .him that cometh to me I will in no wise cast out.

> Verily, verily (truly) I say unto you, He that believeth on me (Christ) hath everlasting life" — (John 6:37, 47).

He also is a righteous God and a God of indignation to those who reject Him. . .

> ". . .he that believeth not is condemned already, because he hath not believed in the name of the only begotten Son of God" — (John 3:18).

> "And whosoever was not found written in the book of life was cast into the lake of fire" — (Revelation 20:15).

YOUR MOST IMPORTANT DECISION IN LIFE

Sin entered the world and God hates sin, yet because God loved us God sent His Son Jesus Christ to die on the cross to pay the price for your sins and mine.

If you place your trust in Him, God will freely forgive you of your sins.

> "For by grace are ye saved through faith; and that not of yourselves: it is the gift of God:

> Not of works, lest any man should boast"—(Ephesians 2:8, 9).

> ". . .He that heareth my word, and believeth on Him that sent me, hath everlasting life, and shall not come into condemnation: but is passed from death unto life" — (John 5:24).

What about you? Have you accepted Christ as your personal Saviour?

Do you realize that right now you can know the reality of this new life in Christ Jesus? Right now you can dispel the doubt that is in your mind concerning your future. Right now you can ask Christ to come into your heart. And right now you can be assured of eternal life in heaven.

All of your riches here on earth — all of your financial security — all of your material wealth, your house, your land will crumble into nothingness in a few years.

And as God has told us:

> "It is appointed unto men once to die, but after this the judgment:
>
> So Christ was once offered to bear the sins of many; and unto them that look for Him shall He appear the second time without sin unto salvation" — (Hebrews 9:27, 28).

Are you willing to sacrifice an eternity with Christ in Heaven for a few years of questionable material gain that will lead to death and destruction? If you do not accept Christ as your personal Saviour, you have only yourself to blame for the consequences.

Or would you right now, as you are reading these very words of this book, like to know without a shadow of a doubt that you are on the road to Heaven — that death is not the end of life but actually the climactic beginning of the most wonderful existence that will ever be — a life with the Lord Jesus Christ and with your friends, your relatives, and your loved ones who have accepted Christ as their Saviour.

It's not a difficult thing to do. So many religions and so many people have tried to make the simple Gospel message of Christ complex. You can not work your way into heaven — heaven is the gift of God to those who believe in Jesus Christ.

HOW TO GET TO HEAVEN

I have met many well-intentioned people who feel that "all roads lead to Heaven." This, unfortunately, is false. *All roads do NOT lead to Heaven.*

All roads lead to DEATH . . . except ONE ROAD and ONE WAY. Jesus

Christt said:

> "I am the door; by me if any man enter in, he shall be
> saved ..."   (John 10:9)

> "He that entereth not by the door into the sheepfold, but
> climbeth up some other way, the same is a thief and a
> robber."   (John 10:1)

There are not many Teachers. There is ONE Teacher, the Lord, Christ
Jesus! There are not many roads. There is ONE ROAD ... the Lord,
Christ Jesus. The Bible warns us:

> "But though we, or an angel from Heaven, preach any other
> gospel unto you than that which we have preached unto you,
> let him be accursed."   (Galatians 1:8)

No matter how great your works — no matter how kind you are — no
matter how philanthropic you are — it means nothing in the sight of
God, because in the sight of God, your riches are as filthy rags.

> "...all our righteousnesses are as filthy rags..." —(Isaiah 64:6).

Christ expects you to come as you are, a sinner, recognizing your need
of a Saviour, the Lord Jesus Christ.

Understanding this, why not bow your head right now and give this
simple prayer of faith to the Lord that is found on the **next page.**

Say it in your own words. It does not have to be a beautiful oratorical
prayer — simply a prayer of humble contrition.

My Personal Decision for CHRIST

"Lord Jesus, I know that I'm a sinner and that I cannot save myself by good works. I believe that you died for me and that you shed your blood for my sins on the cross. I believe that you rose again from the dead. And now I am receiving you as my personal Saviour, my Messiah and Lord, my only hope of salvation. I know that I'm a sinner and deserve God's wrath and judgment. I know that I cannot save myself. Lord, be merciful to me, a sinner, and save me according to the promise of Your Word. I want Christ to come into my heart now to be my Saviour, Lord and Master."

Signed ....

Date ....

"That if thou shalt confess with thy mouth the Lord Jesus, and shalt believe in thine heart that God hath raised Him from the dead, thou shalt be saved.

For whosoever shall call upon the name of the Lord shall be saved." — (Romans 10:9, 13)

If you have signed the above, having just taken Christ as your personal Saviour and Lord . . . I would like to rejoice with you in your new found faith.

Write to me . . . Salem Kirban, Kent Road, Huntingdon Valley, Penna. 19006 . . . and I'll send you a little booklet to help you start living your new life in Christ.

Use this ORDER FORM to order additional copies of

**HOW TO KEEP
HEALTHY and
HAPPY by
FASTING!**

by Salem Kirban

You will want to give **HOW TO
KEEP HEALTHY and HAPPY by
FASTING** to your loved ones and
friends.

An excellent book to give to one
who is ill or having weight problems. The information in this book
could save their life!

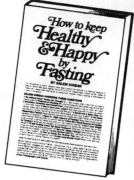

Over 30
PHOTOGRAPHS,
ILLUSTRATIONS
and CHARTS!
Easy-to-read
TYPE!

PRICES

1 copy: $2.95

3 copies: $7.95 (You save .90)
7 copies: 15.95 (You save $4.70)
12 copies: 24.95 (You save $10.45)

WE PAY POSTAGE!

ORDER FORM

**SALEM KIRBAN, Inc.
Kent Road
Huntingdon Valley, Penna. 19006 U.S.A.**

Enclosed find $ _____ for _____ copies of
HOW TO KEEP HEALTHY and HAPPY by FASTING by Salem Kirban.

Ship postage paid to:

Name _____
(PLEASE PRINT)

Street _____

City _____

State _____ Zip Code _____

BOOKS on BETTER HEALTH by ADELLE DAVIS

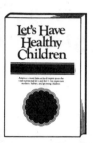

LET'S HAVE HEALTHY CHILDREN
by Adelle Davis

Single copy: $2.00

America's most famous food expert gives the vital nutritional do's and don't for expectant mothers, babies, and growing children. Chapters include:

A Good Diet Brings Rich Rewards
Prepare for Your Baby Before Each Conception
Recognize the Storm Signals
For an Easier Delivery
Maintaining Breast Milk of High Quality
An Easy Method of Baby Feeding
Abnormalities During Early Babyhood
Infections Can Be Avoided
Delay Can Bring Tragedy
Allergies? Why Keep Them?

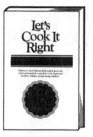

LET'S COOK IT RIGHT
by Adelle Davis

Single copy: $2.25

What are the best ways to prepare food so that it is nutritionally best for you? Adelle Davis reveals her secrets. Chapters include:

You Need Have No Failures in Cooking Meats
Make Delicious Gravies or None at All
Get Acquainted with Fish
Meat Substitutes for Limited Budgets
Serve Eggs and Cheese Daily
Appetizers Contribute to Health
Serve Your Salads First
Soups Are Fun to Make
Keep the Nutritive Value in Your Vegetables
Fortify Your Cereals
Desserts Can Contribute to Health

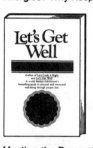

LET'S GET WELL
by Adelle Davis

Single copy: $2.25

Adelle Davis shows how the proper selection of foods and supplements can hasten recovery from illness. A Best Seller! Chapters include:

Meeting the Demands of Stress
Those "Cholesterol" Problems
Heart Attacks, America's Most Lethal Disease
Learn to Live Without an Ulcer
Diabetes Is Not Always Permanent
Arthritis Can Often Be Relieved
Problems of the Digestive System
Allergies are Stress Diseases
Kidney Stones Can Be Dissolved
Problems That Concern Women
Eye Problems and Diseases

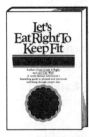

LET'S EAT RIGHT TO KEEP FIT
by Adelle Davis

Single copy: $2.25

Adelle Davis reveals her bestselling guide to physical and emotional well-being through proper diet. 3 Million in Print. Chapters include:

Breakfast Gets the Day's Work Done
One Trick in Staying Young
Are Blue Mondays Necessary?
Study Yourself in the Mirror
Reducing Blood Cholesterol
Nature's Own Tranquilizer
How Firm a Foundation?
Personal Rewards of Good Nutrition
Vitamin E, Needed by Every Cell
Vitamin C Can Protect the Body
Can Vitamin Supplements Meet our Needs?

SALEM KIRBAN, Inc., Kent Rd., Huntingdon Valley, Penna. 19006

Salem Kirban, Inc., Kent Rd., Huntingdon Valley, Penna. 19006

ENTER my order for the books I have checked below. Price includes postage and packing. Enclose check with order.

☐ Let's Have Healthy Children (2.00)   ☐ Let's Cook It Right (2.25)
☐ Let's Get Well (2.25)   ☐ Let's Eat Right to Keep Fit (2.25)

NAME _____

ADDRESS _____

CITY _____ State _____

ZIP

NOW! SAVE MONEY ON FOOD BILLS! ENJOY HEALTH FOOD

LITTLE GREEN ACRE

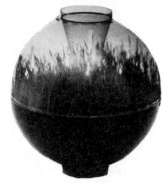

The Beginning of Nutritious, Popular Meals For only PENNIES A DAY!

Did you realize you could have a Garden in just 12 INCHES of space right in your own kitchen?

Imagine having a harvest of nutritious home grown sprouts every 3-4 days!

The chemical additives we use to preserve our food are destroying our health and the cost of medical care is skyrocketing. How can we solve this dilemma? By creating an inexpensive method of producing "healthy" food.

Sprouted seeds, the very beginning of new life, are one of the **highest** forms of nutrition known.

LITTLE GREEN ACRE makes it possible for you to enjoy home grown sprouts for just pennies a day! What a wonderful way to guide and guard your family's health, protect your budget and provide fresh food . . . even in winter!

YOUR GARDEN IN A BOWL

You don't need a degree in agriculture to produce 3 exciting, healthful meals a day at a fraction of your present food budget. The vital nutrition provided by sprouted seeds can now be home grown easily and efficiently!

For the first time, with LITTLE GREEN ACRE, the elements needed to produce sprouts: light, humidity and air circulation, are in balanced harmony.

The Little Green Acre grows sprouts which are tender, sweet and green with chlorophyll; just like spinach, lettuce and endive directly from the garden.

The colorful sphere is specifically designed to utilize those light rays in the spectrum which enhance sprout growth. And, as a decorative addition to any room in your home, sprouting for food and fun provides a garden of delights for children and is an adventure for the entire family!

To Protect Your Family
SPROUTS PROVIDE YOUR HIGHEST VITAMIN CONTENT
Naturally!

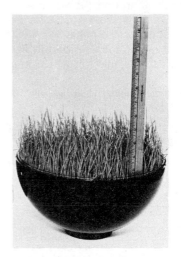

Sprouts are actually described as "perfect" because all the life-giving proteins, carbohydrates, oils, vitamins and minerals necessary to support our life system are stored within the seed itself.

When seeds begin to sprout, their vitamin content accelerates at a remarkable rate. The first shoots of soybeans (per 100 grams of seed) contain about 100 milligrams of vitamin C, but after 72 hours the content soars to approximately 700 milligrams, an increase of almost 700 percent! **This means that soybean sprouts contain almost 20 times the amount of vitamin C that is provided in a glass of orange juice!** Similar comparisons can be made for most of the vitamins, including Vitamin A, the B vitamins and E.

Sprouts satisfy one's need for protein without consuming high calories. One ounce of meat, both lean and fat, contains approximately 80 calories . . . whereas one ounce of beansprouts has only about 10 calories and . . . contains no cholesterol!

SALEM KIRBAN, INC.
2117 Kent Road, Huntingdon Valley, Pennsylvania 19006

BOOKS ON HEALTH by PAUL C. BRAGG

Paul C. Bragg is himself the best testimonial for the value of his teachings. He is a great-great-grandfather and has authored over 30 books. His books are read by thousands around the world, and his teachings are followed by famous people such as Billy Graham, Doris Day, Conrad Hilton and Jack LaLanne. Gloria Swanson was one of his first health students. Paul C. Bragg is a physical therapist and a giant in the field of nutrition, health and physical fitness. For over 40 years he has counselled Kings, Queens, Politicians, Sportsmen and Statesmen.

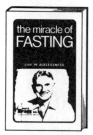

THE MIRACLE OF FASTING
by Paul C. Bragg
Single copy: $3.25
In 33 inspiring chapters, Paul Bragg reveals new discoveries about an old miracle for agelessness, physical, mental and spiritual rejuvenation. Interesting highlights include his own experiences in fasting.

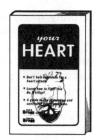

HOW TO KEEP YOUR HEART HEALTHY AND FIT
by Paul C. Bragg
Single copy: $2.25
Are you a candidate for a heart attack? Learn how to fight this No. 1 killer! You will find this book a guide to the prevention and control of heart problems. Well worth the price!

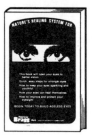

PREPARING FOR MOTHERHOOD NATURE'S WAY
by Paul C. Bragg
Single copy: $2.25
An excellent guidebook for the mother-to-be and for the mother. You will find everything from proper prenatal exercises to proper nutrition for your baby and for you. A must for every mother!

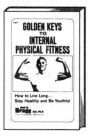

GOLDEN KEYS TO INTERNAL PHYSICAL FITNESS
by Paul C. Bragg
Single copy: $2.25
This book tells you how to live long, stay healthy and be youthful! Life can begin (or end) at 40. If you are starting to feel sluggish at 40, 50 or 60, this book will reveal how you can be internally fit!

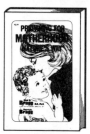

NATURE'S HEALING SYSTEM FOR BETTER EYESIGHT REGARDLESS OF AGE
Single copy: $1.25
This book will open your eyes to better vision. It will show you how your eyes can heal themselves and how to keep your eyes sparkling and youthful. Quick, easy steps!

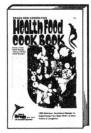

HEALTH FOOD COOKBOOK
by Paul C. Bragg
Single copy: $4.25
Here you will find 1000 of the world's finest health recipes! Recipes to supercharge your body with youthful vitality and longevity! Plus Herb Charts, Vitamin-Mineral Charts and Weight Control Menus.

SALEM KIRBAN Books on Prophecy

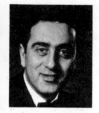

Salem Kirban is a graduate of Girard College and received his Bachelor of Science at Temple University at Philadelphia. He is married. He and his wife, Mary, have 5 children.

In the last 5 years he has written over 20 bestselling books. GUIDE TO SURVIVAL, 666 and I PREDICT have each sold over 1/4 MILLION copies!

Many of his titles are sold through bookstores by Moody Press and Tyndale House/Publishers. However, you can use this ORDER FORM to order your books DIRECT by mail.

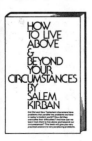

HOW TO LIVE ABOVE and BEYOND YOUR CIRCUMSTANCES
by Salem Kirban

Single copy: $3.95

At last! Practical answers to perplexing problems that face Christians everyday. A new book that is refreshingly *different*. Whatever your problems . . . here's a book that can change your life . . . for the better!

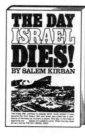

THE DAY ISRAEL DIES
by Salem Kirban

Single copy: $ $2.95

The 6-Day War, contrary to popular belief, never ended! One day, in the midst of agonizing war... peace will suddenly come. When this day does arrive it will be THE DAY ISRAEL DIES!

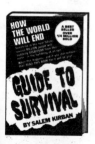

GUIDE TO SURVIVAL
by Salem Kirban

Single copy: $2.95
3 copies: $ 5
10 copies: $15

This book tells you how the world will END! Almost 300 pages. Over 50 photos and charts! Over 1/2 MILLION SOLD!

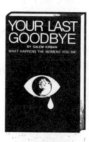

YOUR LAST GOODBYE
by Salem Kirban

Single copy: $3.95

The Book that tells you all about HEAVEN and exactly what happens THE MOMENT YOU DIE. Over 65 charts and photos. FULL COLOR. Over 300 pages.

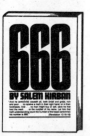

666
by Salem Kirban

Single copy: $2.95

A suspenseful novel on the Tribulation Period. 666 is a novel which vividly captures events as they may happen. Over 275 pages. Over 50 PHOTOGRAPHS and illustrations.

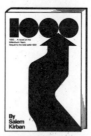

1000
by Salem Kirban

Single copy: $ 2.95
3 copies: $ 7

SEQUEL to the best seller 666! Weaves the same plausable characters into the prophesied events of the MILLENNIUM Period. Over 50 photographs and charts.

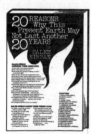

20 REASONS
WHY THIS PRESENT EARTH MAY NOT LAST ANOTHER 20 YEARS

Single copy: $ 2.95

Ecology, new events, alignment of nations plus other signs of the times indicate we are living in perilous times. Book sets no dates but reveals how close we are to Rapture.

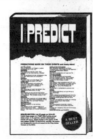

I PREDICT
by Salem Kirban

Single copy: $ 2.95
3 copies: $ 7

Now! The book that dares to reveal the disasters of the future. Filled with photographs and charts. Sealed section with Timetable of Events!